HOW TO BE HAPPY, HEALTHY … AND HOT

SVEN REBEL was born in 1970, went to school in Berlin, Kreuzberg, and after several wild years in Cologne, Paris, London, and San Francisco, returned to Berlin in 2000, where he lives now. For over fifteen years, Sven Rebel has created news reports, documentaries, and shows for German television. Today, he is a successful life coach, spotting trends and offering advice on how to create an individual lifestyle and optimize one's personal choices. In private, his interests revolve around fast cars, motorcycles, and the good life.

Sven Rebel's *Joyful Gay Sex* was published by Bruno Gmünder.

Sven Rebel

How to Be Happy, Healthy ... and Hot

The Ultimate Gay Lifestyle Guide

BRUNO GMÜNDER

Disclaimer: The photographs published in this book should not be understood to indicate the sexual orientation of the models shown in them.

HOW TO BE HAPPY, HEALTHY ... AND HOT

Copyright © 2014 Bruno Gmünder Verlag GmbH
Kleiststraße 23-26, D-10787 Berlin
info@brunogmuender.com

Text: © 2010/20014 Sven Rebel
Original Title: Von Mann zu Mann
Translation: Nicola Heine

Cover design: Steffen Kawelke
Layout: Dolph Caesar
Cover photos: © Falcon Studios
Models: Aden and Jordan Jaric
www.falconstudios.com

Photos:
© Falcon Studios, www.FalconStudios.com:
6, 9, 13, 14, 20, 25, 26, 34, 45, 47, 49, 52, 65, 69, 70, 77, 81, 93, 96, 105, 116, 132, 134, 137, 141, 161, 172, 177, 181, 184
© Lucas Entertainment, www.LucasEntertainment.com:
10, 23, 67, 89, 94, 149, 153, 157, 174, 179
© Ralf Rühmeier, www.ralfruehmeier.de:
100, 117-129, 185
istockphoto.com:
16, 28, 31, 33, 41, 57, 72, 85, 98, 103, 109, 110, 112, 113, 115, 131, 147, 155, 169, 170
© C1R, www.c1r.com:
143

Printed in South Korea
ISBN: 978-3-86787-693-3

More about our books and authors:
www.brunogmuender.com

For my man

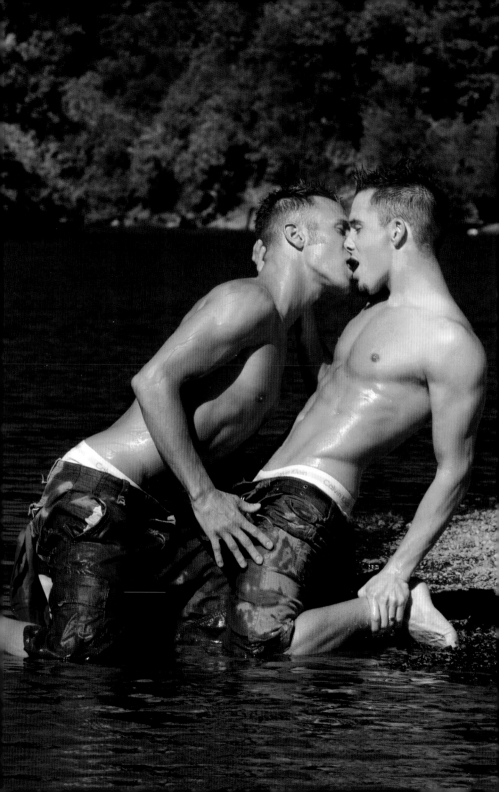

Contents

Who Was Gay?
A Real Man
The Bogus Man

Which Screenings Should a Gay Man Have?

But Why Can't Men Just Use the Same Creams Women Do?
Detox—Spring Cleaning from the Inside
Detox—The Terrible Truth
Exfoliating—New Skin, New Me
How Much Grooming Does a Man Need?
Bald Is Beautiful
How to Shave Your Head
Dat Ass!
Hands—Sticky Fingers
Injectable Beauty—The Botox Myth

How to Get a Proper Tan—Time to Get Out the Grill
How to Get Really Tan
The Right Fragrance
A Good Suit—Nice Threads

Contents

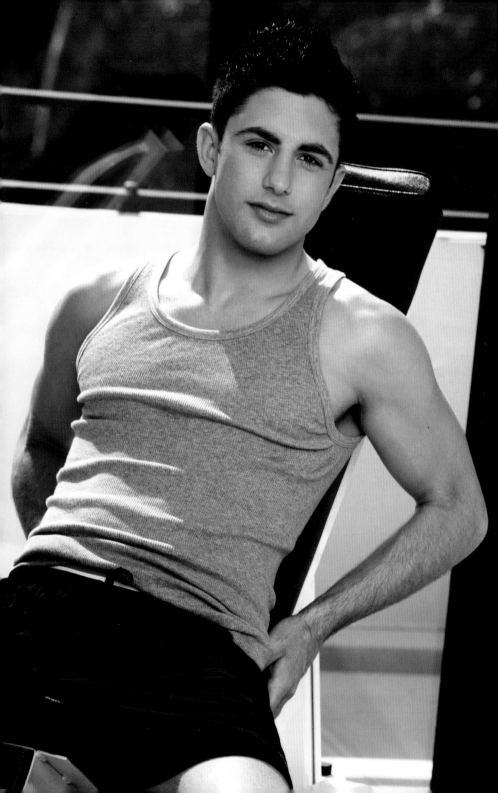

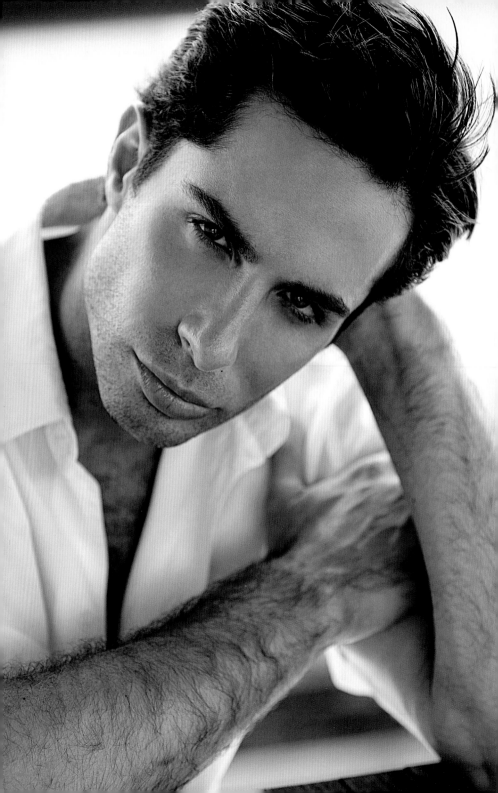

Introduction

For some time now, there have been any number of books on the mar-ket in which various learned writers inform their gentle readers that they are not real men unless they are able to, say, land a Boeing plane at the drop of a hat. To be perfectly honest, if I should ever find myself in a plane that, for whatever reason, is not equipped with a fully functional pilot, I really couldn't care less who gets the thing onto the ground safely—be it a swashbuckling adventurer bursting with testosterone or a busty blonde lady. As long as they get me down in one piece, I really couldn't give a damn about their masculinity. Changing tires is another case in point, generally seen as the domain of the real man. Why? All I can say is: Real men have moved on; once they've realized that almost any woman is just as capable of doing it, they will (politely) give way to here. Let the girls get their hands dirty as well—all in the name of equality, of course. In addition, the authors of these books, apparently laboring under a crippling lack of self-confidence, insist on the importance of knowing how to join the foreign legion, how to become pope, or finally learn how to stay awake during sex.

All I can say is: Straight men of the world, cast your eyes upon your gay brothers! The word "sleep" has no meaning for them if there is an opportunity for good sex within a thirty-mile radius.

Gay men, it would seem, are less burdened by their masculinity. If the subject is the Foreign Legion, all they think about is an intense session with one of those hot soldiers. If it's a Boeing 747, they will fantasize about joining the Mile High Club. And if you're talking about the Pope, every gay man's thoughts will turn immediately to those cute guys in the Swiss Guard.

Let's put it this way: While your average heterosexual man is still arguing about Cristiano Ronaldo's abilities on the soccer field, most red-blooded gay men will have already been masturbating to photos of him in the nude. Real men of action!

Where am I going with all this? Quite simply: Even the most effeminate gay man tends to just live out his masculinity, whereas straight men have to read a book to find out how to compensate for their unfulfilled fantasies!

Sadly enough, there is more to life than just sex, and you need to know more than how to perform an anal douche properly if you want to be at your best at all times and successfully navigate your way through everyday life.

Now that I have already written everything there is to know about sex in my excellent *Joyful Gay Sex* (this is, of course, a totally objective assessment), the following book presents a handy guide to the good gay life. Here you will find everything you need to know to look good in any situation and to be able to enjoy your gay lifestyle to the fullest.

This is a book to help you to gracefully soar above the larger and smaller pitfalls of everyday life, a book that transcends useless clichés and stereotypes and instead provides solid advice and instructions that anyone can follow—if he wants to! A book ... that is hetero-inclusive! So, go ahead and give a copy to all of your straight friends—it definitely won't hurt them!

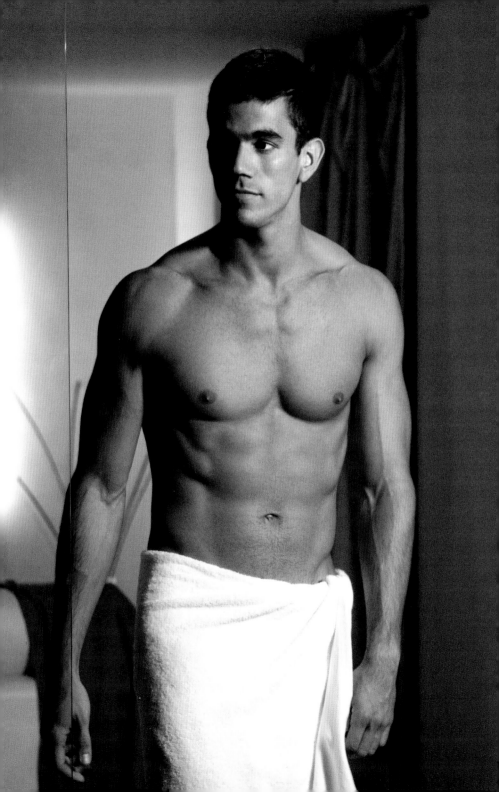

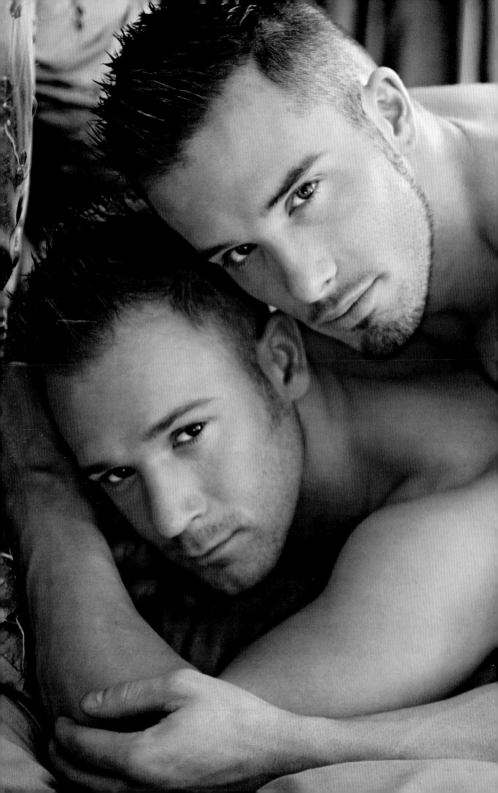

Lifestyle

What is the most important skill every gay man should have mastered? That's right: small talk! Whether you're chatting someone up, or at work, at a fancy dinner, or in a hip bar—if you can interject a witty comment or two into the conversation, you'll not only make yourself agreeable, you'll also be able to keep even the most difficult conversation going. That's why I have included a number of light "interludes" in this book, listing a couple of uselessly useful facts. Just memorize these, and you'll be the star of every conversation!

Gay Lifestyle
It is a proven fact that gay men live better than breeders! Forty-three percent of all gay men spend most of their money on vacations, while only twenty-nine percent of all straight men do. Exclusive gentlemen's wear is important to twenty-three percent of all gay men, ten percent more than straight men.

Young, Chic, and Gay
Yves Saint Laurent is considered by many to be the perfect example of the successful gay man who lives his life in style. After all, he was Christian Dior's assistant at the age of seventeen, the youngest couturier of all time. Although he was outlived by his archrival Karl Lagerfeld, the general agreement in the world of fashion is that the former ponytail-wearer will never outshine him. The two of them presumably represent the prototype of gay cat fighting!

Excuse Me?
Arnold Schwarzenegger has come a long way. But he still can't express himself too clearly. Money quote: "I think that gay marriage is something that should be between a man and a woman."

We Are Not Alone
It is assumed that one in ten people are homosexual. But that's nothing compared to sea horses. A third of them are gay!

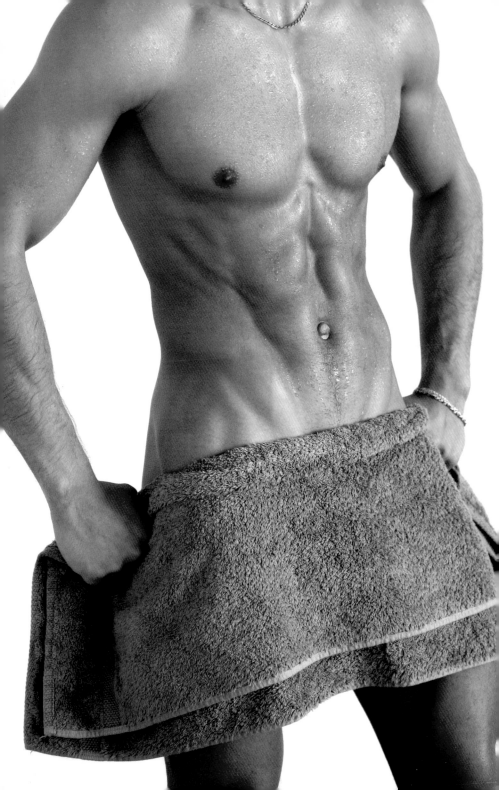

Gay? What You Need to Know

Why a book for gay men? Why can't they just read a guide for *all* men? Why do they need special treatment? Quite simple! Gays are men too, but they are different from straight men. You don't believe me? Well, here are some facts on the topic!

Are you born gay or is gayness a learned quality? This question has been the subject of scientific debate for many years. Now science has finally produced some halfway solid results: Researchers in Sweden comprehensively analyzed 7,600 sets of twins. They found out that seven percent of them had had sex with a same-sex partner at least once. The analysis showed that seventeen percent of the time, family and societal norms had a slight influence on their choice. But for considerably more men, eighteen to thirty-nine percent, their genetic makeup was the main contributing factor to their gay agenda. But it is neither your family nor your genetic makeup that have the greatest influence on sexual orientation. It is your own personal experiences, be they positive or negative, and these can be a factor even before birth. Isn't that a wonderful result? It shows that gay men are not simply a single group among men, but also that there is a different reason for each one of them—and a different path of life, just the same as for everyone else. Surely that is the best reason to rejoice in your own individuality and live just as your heart—and, of course, your cock—desires!

But does being gay fulfill a purpose? Of course! Not only has the cause of homosexuality been the subject of intensive research, but also the "why?" Mother Nature would hardly haul any kind of development around for thousands of years if it didn't make any sense—evolution does not forgive a mistake!

One explanation that science has to offer, and one I find particularly pleasing, is that gay men form the missing link between the sexes. In a nutshell, the theory says that because gay men are generally unable to reproduce, their life energy is channeled into society as a whole, and is not focused selfishly on preserving their own offspring. To put it another way:

The gay man as such, while being a real man, is no stranger to feminine ways of thinking! Doesn't that sound like an improvement on the standard gender model? No wonder there's so much homophobia around, They're just jealous!

The Spartans, a people no one in their right mind would accuse of being effeminate, did things completely differently. Gay men were the most popular and the best warriors among the Spartans, as they had no familial duties and could be more ruthless and selfless in battle.

I may be going out on a philosophical limb by adhering to this theory, but to me it all sounds quite reasonable.

Who Was Gay?

There have been plenty of smart gays around, even before I came along. Or to put it differently: The world would be a much less pleasant place without gay men! So, here is my personal top ten list of historically relevant homos—from the past to the present!

TOP TEN LIST OF WHO WAS GAY

10 The first official gay man was a pharaoh: Akhenaten. And as befits a true homo, he was famous for his sense of beauty and his exquisite taste. And just in passing, he was the first to guide religious faith from polytheism to a belief in one god, even though this monotheist intermezzo was only a short-lived one. Another interesting fact is that the queen reigning at his side was also to achieve world fame—for seated on the throne beside him was none other than the lovely Nefertiti!

9 Another gay man was one of the most important philosophers ever: good old Socrates, who still influences Western thought today and was the first to espouse the concept of persuading your opponent by using facts rather than force. Plato's teacher was presumably delighted to live in ancient Greece, where pederasty was a popular pastime.

8 The mightiest general and conqueror of them all, Alexander the Great, was as gay as it gets. However, the real Alexander bore absolutely no similarity to the peroxide-blond Colin Farrell in the terrible historical epic "Alexander"—the original article was probably more of a macho brute.

7 Another general, Julius Caesar, murdered by Brutus, demonstrably enjoyed the occasional nookie with other guys. Which throws a totally new light on conditions within the legions …

6 And, of course, Leonardo da Vinci, perhaps the greatest genius of all time, was also gay! No need for further elaboration!

5 And in case you've ever wondered why the famous ceiling fresco in the Sistine Chapel features so many naked and muscular men … that's right: Michelangelo was gay, too!

4 Another genius we can proudly point to in our gay honor roll is Alexander von Humboldt. He was the first scientist to come up with the idea of a network, merging the humanities and the natural sciences to foster a new way of thinking outside the box.

3 + 3.5 We have the one-hundred-percent-gay Peter Tchaikovsky to thank for beautiful pieces of music. The American president Abraham Lincoln wasn't always on point, but he did have a four-year affair with a cute guy.

2 If you hear a German say "My dick's as hard as Krupp's steel," then small wonder. The inventor and industrial giant Friedrich Alfred Krupp was also quite an enthusiastic admirer of his own gender.

1 And thus the list continues up to the present day, to one man who with a single sentence did more for gay acceptance than any number of politicians in any political organization. I'm talking about Klaus Wowereit, the mayor of Berlin, who famously said, "I'm gay, and it's fine that way!"

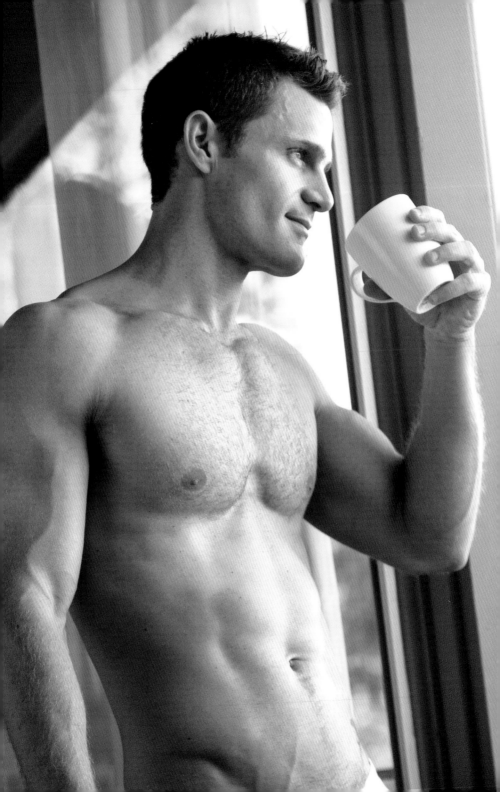

A Real Man

Let's be frank here: Visually, it isn't that hard to look like a real man—after all, we're all familiar with the clichés. But real masculinity is rarely defined as having big muscles or a hairy belly. Pretty much anyone would be disappointed if this kind of visual miracle were to open his mouth and all your illusions were to crumble to dust because it turns out that your hot Ken is a lot more like a hot mess of a Barbie.

At the end of the day, it's our subconscious mind that decides whether or not we see guys as really masculine. And then it's really the finer details that turn the boys into real men.

So let's get started with this topic—with my own personal, completely subjective top five unmistakable signs of real manliness! Feel free to follow these examples!

TOP FIVE REAL MEN ...

5 ... can park with one hand
Men are demonstrably better at parking a car than women are—although there are a couple of girls who do quite well at it. That's why the boys need to step up their game if they want to keep their gender-specific edge. I would recommend that the gay boys especially turn the following exercise into an effective part of their own lifestyle: Learn to park with one hand! This means nothing other than casually backing into even the narrowest parking space in three easy steps, with one hand on the wheel and the other on the stick shift—without constantly changing your grip, hectically engaging the clutch, or nervously glancing back and forth. Who wouldn't go weak in the knees at such an exhibition of perfect spatial abilities? Just a small gift with a great effect! Doesn't any girl or guy who takes five minutes to parallel park into an enormous space—with the help of random passers-by or while frantically cranking at the wheel all the while—lose a couple of points in the race to our hearts? A classic example of how to be awarded oodles of man-points from onlookers with the most inconspicuous of actions!

4 ... are bow-legged
Even though bowlegs are commonly sneered at as a semi-disability, there can surely be no bodily feature that tells you so clearly that its owner has played a lot of soccer during his youth. And that kind of guy has got to be a real man! While many gay men stalk about with straight knee joints and tensed ass cheeks in imitation of a bad model on the catwalk, a bow-legged

man always walks casually. And without even trying, he is the embodiment of coolness.

No wonder the cowboys of the legendary Old West always adopted a broad-legged gait! So boys, give us less of the ballerina and more of the cowboy's amble.

3 ... are brutes in suits

I'm assuming most of you are already aware of the enormous swath that even the most average of men in a well-fitting suit can cut in general—and when flirting in particular. (If you haven't tried it yet, take a look at my guidelines for the perfect suit later on in this book!) But what's even hotter than just a good suit is when you get to see the real brute lurking underneath the natty three-piece. You can't get more confident than a vulgar tattoo peeking provocatively out of a shirtsleeve or above the collar line. You can tell from a thousand yards away that all things vanilla are completely foreign to this man and that you'll need about two weeks of rest after a night with him. Isn't that hot? After all, the surprise waiting for you after you unwrap him is the best part!

2 ... taste like an ashtray

I think we can all agree that there's nothing hot about bad breath. Nor about cigarette smoke or the stink of alcohol—even though the two of them combined can be a real stimulant. Standing around in a sleazy bar, meeting up with a hot guy, talking with him all evening, drinking beer, getting hotter and hotter for him, followed by—finally—that first kiss with the taste of smoke and beer. Could anything be hotter? This is only sexy in a guy. Just imagine a peroxide blonde woman all decked out in expensive clothes and a Wonderbra whose kisses taste of cigarettes and beer: It just doesn't fit. I'm sorry, dear straight readers, but you're missing out on a real sensual experience here!

1 ... have good manners

The one thing that separates the men from the boys—and which one can easily learn—is good manners! Gay men in particular are frequently lacking in these, believing that they need to be especially bitchy, cynical, or derogatory in order to stand out. They couldn't be more wrong! That's what we call a "fag" or "pissy queen", in the most positive light we might call him a "prole" (as in "proletarian"). A well-mannered guy, on the other hand, is popular and sought-after and is more readily seen as a "real man." And what's not to love? So please, mind your manners. And what you don't know, you can find out by reading this book! It's that easy!

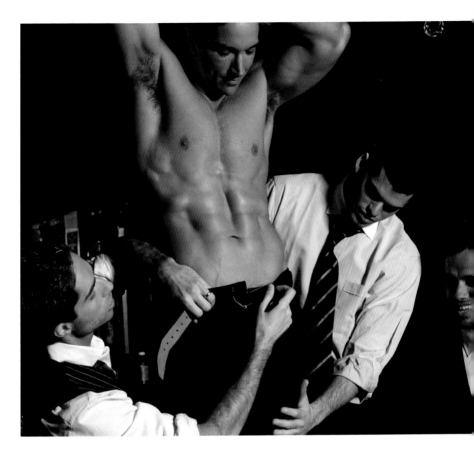

The Bogus Man

And then there are the worst kind of frauds among men. Biologically, their chromosomes place them firmly within the male sex, but there are unmistakable signs that deep inside they feel quite differently. And I don't mean the notorious floppy wrist or the sashaying swing of the hip performed by an ostensible man. Oh, no. For no matter how campy a guy is, he can still be a pretty convincing man! But there are some things that will pulverize any semblance of masculinity within a split second. So, if you don't want to downgrade yourself to girliness, you need to watch the following points so that you don't end up on my hardly objective list of the top five most unmanly behaviors!

5 ... eat soy?

Contrary to the old cliché, real men do not drink only whiskey and beer. The only people to get completely hammered these days are kids whenever they hear the words "all-you-can-drink." Real men, on the other hand, also drink non-alcoholic beverages, and occasionally even milk. But in the last few years, yummy milk pumped from an udder has lost ground with the environmentally- and health-conscious man, giving way to its vegan cousin, soy milk. A pity! Because these boys are not doing themselves any favors. Only softies drink soy milk, and if they aren't soft yet, they will be if they drink enough of it. For soy contains so much female estrogen that a regular and ample consumption can make even the most athletic boys grow lovely soft breasts. I'm not kidding! In the United States, serious athletes avoid all soy products like the plague. But there's even worse news: Researchers at Harvard University have found out that men who eat a lot of soy products suffer a drastic decrease in sperm production. So, it's better not to risk it!

TOP FIVE
REAL MEN
NEVER ...

4 ... bare their midriffs?

Some clothes look adorable on little boys and girls—as long as they're under six years of age. These definitely include cropped T-shirts. Even though overweight girls in low-cut pants and gay men of every age will happily present their midriffs at every opportunity during the height of summer, these shirts are the worst. At best, you might be able to get away with wearing one if you're part of an over-the-hill troop of entertainers at the Jumbo Center on Gran Canaria. It doesn't matter whether you've got rock-hard abs or a wobbly apron of fat—keep it covered. In any case, the older the wearer of a crop top, the shittier the effect. I'm sorry to sound harsh here, but you really needing to start dressing properly. Sometimes more actually is more!

3 ... like Madonna?

How can gay men still possibly be into Madonna? Whatever her achievements over the past years, now that she's turned into an emaciated lump of cartilage, surely she stands for everything today's gay man should want to avoid—a buzz killing, old, frustrated non-person, still on the hunt for young men. What makes the whole thing even worse is her feeble stabs at remaining relevant with the occasional outpouring of dull, esoteric gobbledygook. She serves as a warning to every gay man over forty who, despite his age, would never dream of looking that desperate and really just wants to have some fun in life. She has brought about the destruction of her own legacy. Don't we all have fond memories of the revolutionary Madonna who showed us all that you can achieve anything you set your heart on? It's a real shame!

2 ... follow a mass trend?

It is a universally acknowledged fact that gays are total trendsetters! Before anything reaches the media, gay boys have generally already heard all about it. Another fact is that men love electronic gadgets. The newer and the more sophisticated, the better. Then what in the world is half of the homo world doing, wandering about with those little white iPods? They look like your granddad's hearing aid! What's worse is that half the gay community have paid loads of cash for the privilege of destroying their otherwise highly-prized individuality. There are plenty of much better, nicer looking and cheaper MP3 players on the market now that don't keep you tied to one and the same download portal. Wake up, gay men—rise up and take back your roles as trailblazers!

1 ... wear "sexy" underwear?

Commercials tend to give you the impression that men are really into brightly colored and bizarrely-patterned underwear. This is incorrect. According to what most leading chain stores say, leopard print underpants, transparent briefs, or boxer shorts with elephant trunks are for the most part bought by elderly fat heterosexuals who are all single—and with good reason. Rent boys, strippers, and go-go boys buy them too, but in this case we're talking about professional wear. A real gay man will wear nice white briefs such as those made fashionable by Calvin Klein many years ago, or boxer shorts of the kind that peek out over the jeans of hot young skaters. The worst are those panties that boast a sophisticated system that will make your package look bigger or pull your ass tighter. This is simply cheating the end consumer. Real men are proud of their dicks, for no matter what size it is, its owner will always have fun with it—and anyone who starts out trying to disguise what's in his pants will only end up with a pretty large complex! So, steer clear!

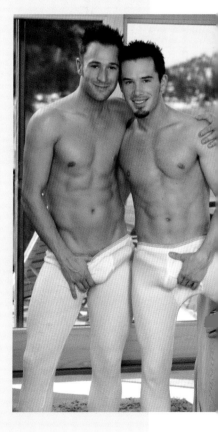

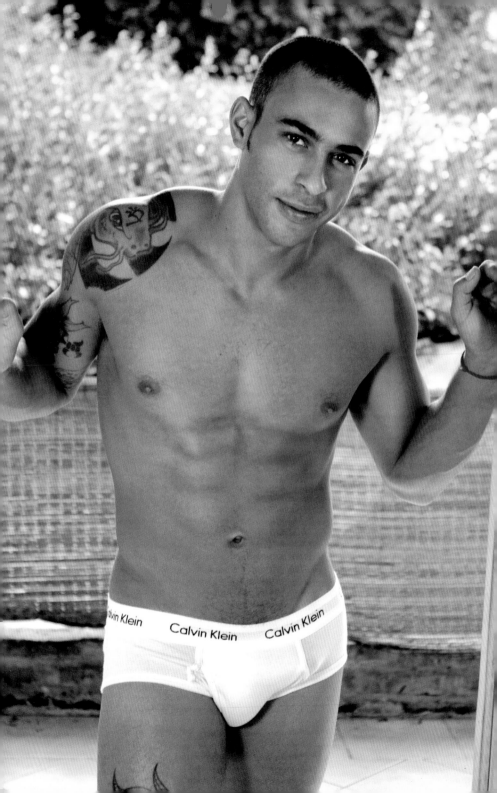

Men – Facts and Figures

More concrete facts so that you'll never be lacking for a smart comment during any bout of small-talk.

Stubble
Now that the full beard has become fashionable once again, we report the following information: The face of the average man has all of 25,000 hair follicles.

Wetlands
An adult male will lose an incredible fifteen liters of perspiration per day doing heavy labor. Let's hope he has a deodorant on him.

Hot Air
The temperature of an average man's fart is 98.6°F. It moves at a velocity of nearly three meters per second. This happens about fourteen times per day on average—probably the actual culprit for global warming.

Going Down
According to a study of the Indiana University at Bloomington, oral sex keeps you young at heart, but only if you're gay. The most orally active gay men are in the 50+ age group. For straight men, giving oral sex (to women!) plummets after 40.

Gold 'n' Locks
In 2013, throughout the world, 1.87 billion dollars were spent on surgical hair restoration—of course mainly by men.

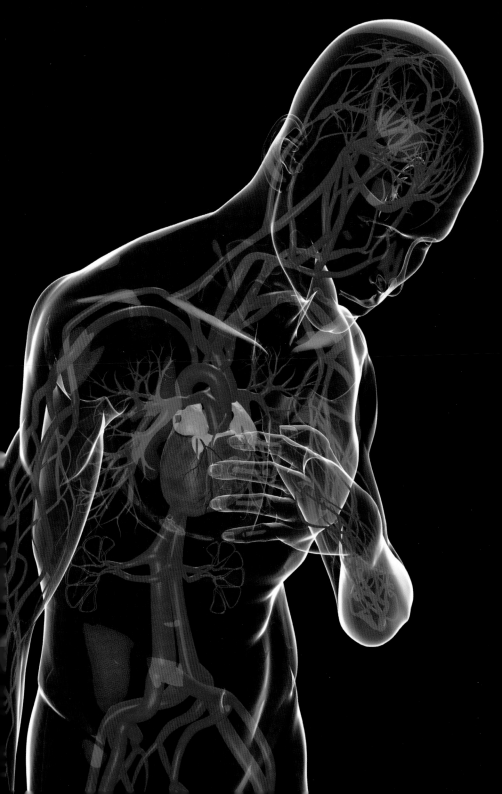

Your Health — A Serious Business

Let's not deceive ourselves. Life is not just an endless series of great events, elegant cocktail parties, and intense dates. There's some revolting disease lurking around every other corner, just waiting to mess with us. The number one cause of death among men is still cardiovascular disease, followed closely by an array of cancerous diseases and all kinds of nasty infections. But there is no need to surrender helplessly to Mother Nature's ruthless selection processes. Regular check-ups can save you a lot of trouble.

Gay men unfortunately need slightly more rigorous check-ups than their heterosexual brothers. This is mainly due to the assortment of sexually transmitted infections (STIs) that plague the gay community. But there is a silver lining for anyone who's not having enough sex. At least that way, you'll have a man in a white coat shoving something up your ass on a regular basis!

Which Screenings Should a Gay Man Have?

Always
The most important screening for a gay man should take place as soon as he becomes sexually active—the HIV test. This test should be repeated regularly, several times a year, depending on how promiscuous you are. Always remember: Having unprotected sex once is enough to get you infected.

Age Twenty-Five and Older
Gay men should have their lymph nodes checked on a regular basis, as some less easily detectable STIs can lead to swellings in typical regions of the body. They don't necessarily have to be dangerous diseases, but they all have to be treated. These screenings are especially advisable for gay men, as some diseases are really prevalent in the gay community.

Every gay man should also have his anal region checked on a yearly basis. This will ensure that genital warts, injuries, hemorrhoids, and anal fissures can be detected quickly. This check-up is vital to a gay man's physical health!

Straight men will only need these check-ups if any problems arise in this area, as they rarely have anyone rarely playing around with their anuses—the poor bastards.

Age Thirty-Five and Older

Every two years you should have the so-called "thirty-five" check-up, which is designed to detect high blood pressure, cardiovascular disease, and metabolic disorders as soon as possible. This is done by creating a risk-profile, undergoing a thorough physical examination, and testing blood and urine for kidney disease, bacterial infections, diabetes, and malnutrition.

And every two years you should have yourself screened for skin cancer. As the number of people affected by this disease is on the rise, you should definitely get this test done. The doctor will inspect your entire body, from your scalp to the deepest skin folds for any suspicious signs.

Age Forty and Older

Now it's time to have your eyes checked and your risk for a heart attack assessed every two years. You have also reached the age when an annual cancer screening can save your life. This means having your external genitalia, your prostrate, and regional lymph nodes examined thoroughly.

Age Fifty and Older

And now it's time for an annual screening for intestinal cancer. You can undergo a real or virtual colonoscopy. In addition, your stool will be checked for hidden traces of blood.

Age Sixty and Older

Last but not least, regular screenings for osteoporosis should form part of your medical check-up schedule.

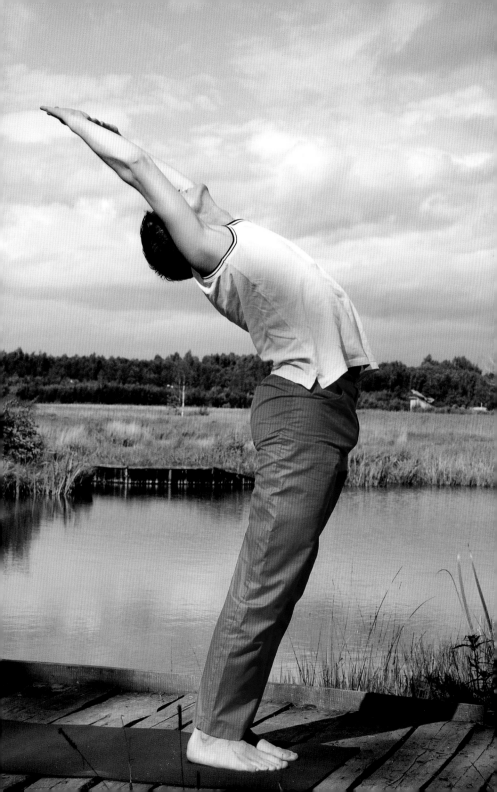

And What Else?

By the way, your medical prevention plan should also include regular trips to the dentist so you can keep your seductive smile.

If you occasionally feel a bit depressed or just not quite up to scratch, or if you feel your virility ebbing, a testosterone test can be helpful. Sometimes you just don't have quite enough male hormones, and just a small extra dose can make you feel sensationally fit again.

Vaccines

I'm not going to talk about basic inoculations here. You should have those in any case. If you're not sure, definitely talk to your doctor. Vaccinating against hepatitis and streptococcus pneumonia is essential for gay guys. I also strongly advise that you get vaccinated against HPV, the Human papillomavirus. This affects about ninety percent of the gay community, but hardly anyone is aware of it. HPV can cause genital warts and, in extreme cases, penile cancer. The problem with the vaccination, however, is that it is only effective when given to very young men, before first sexual contact. But once you have already been infected by the virus, the vaccine can at least protect you from re-infection.

It's Healthy to Blow Your Wad

Good to know—shooting your load is good for your health! A man should ejaculate at least five times a week. For during ejaculation, your prostate, seminal vesicles, and urethra are flushed out and any harmful substances are removed. Research has shown that a man who ejaculates twenty-one times per month has a third less chance of contracting prostate cancer than men who only climax four to seven times per month.

But getting fucked is good for your health too. It can help prevent prostate cancer. There are no solid studies on the topic (who would finance them?), but most proctologists agree that men who get fucked up the ass on a regular basis suffer less from disorders of the prostate. The explanation given for this is that, in addition to hot baths, direct or indirect prostate massages are recommended for patients suffering from prostatitis, as this can relax and soothe the prostate. And that's exactly what happens during anal intercourse: The prostate is given a thorough massage, preventing infections from taking hold or spreading.

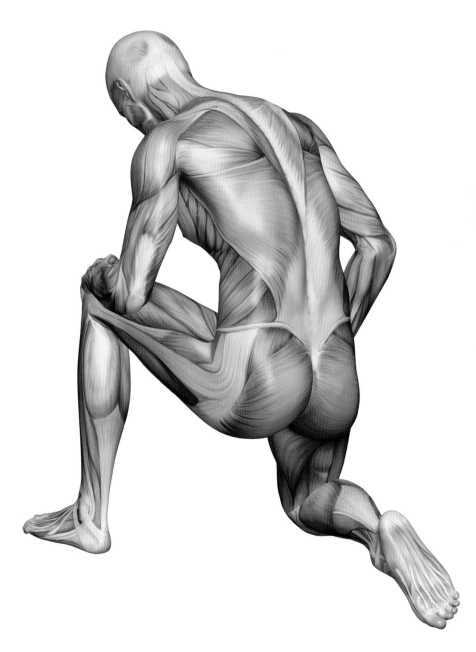

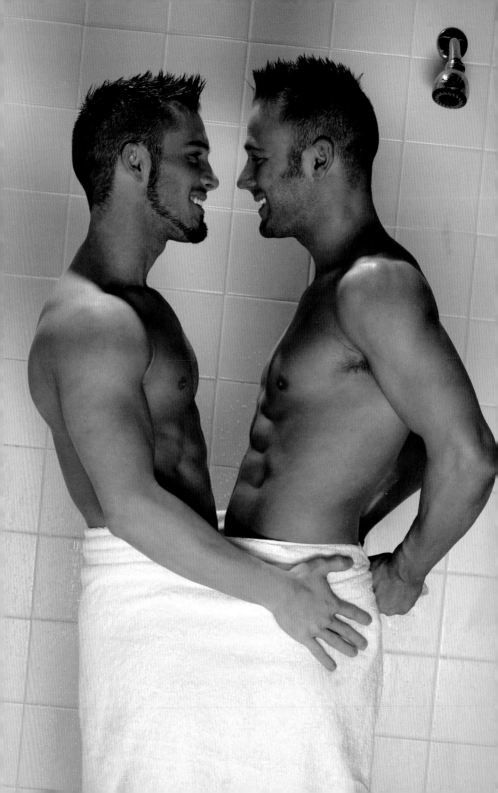

Beauty Queen

Gay men have always taken slightly more care with their appearance than straight men, and have started many a beauty trend. The revelation that good looks can improve your success rate has by now percolated through the entire world of men, and gays are no longer automatically at an advantage during job interviews, for example. Sixty-four percent of all men are convinced that they are perceived as being more successful if they pay more attention to their looks. And that is certainly the case, for—as scientific studies have demonstrated—attractiveness is rewarded. Obviously a well-groomed appearance will grant you a higher success rate in the race for the heart of a sexy guy than looking like a homeless person will. But I'm not talking about the hysterically overgroomed metrosexual. This was a passing fashion trend, instigated by a pretty hot soccer player. But now that most guys have realized that no amount of styling and tweaking will turn them into a Beckham-clone, this wave has already subsided of its own accord.

The rule is: Good masculine grooming is never overpowering! It should always be about making the best of what you have, highlighting your own best qualities, and not about using cosmetics to create another identity for yourself.

You need to be able to feel comfortable in your body and with the care you give it.

You should be enjoying yourself! Because if you spend more time in front of the mirror than you do at work, you'll soon lose interest in personal grooming.

That's why the following pages will supply you with a few solid tips for men to get into better shape visually, according to their own individual desires. Just experiment a little. Find out what works for you and what doesn't. But there's one iron rule: any hairs growing out of your nose and ears must be removed. I don't care how you do it, just get rid of them!

For several years now, I've been writing men's beauty tips for a variety of magazines. During this time, I quickly came to realize that the industry tries to palm all kinds of garbage off on us boys to make us feel prettier. All I can say is: Don't fall for the same tricks the girls have been swallowing for years! As I've said, grooming is a good thing, but only as long as you feel comfortable with it. Be natural in everything you do. Men should always look like men—and not like female impersonators!

But Why Can't Men Just Use the Same Creams Women Do?

They can, and sometimes that's a good thing. Because often enough, you'll find products that are marketed towards men, even though they are essentially the same as women's products, only more expensive and more heavily perfumed. We can all do without these products (I hope you all realize that I can't name any brand names here ...)

As a rule, however, men do need special grooming products. Their skin is different from women's skin. It's thicker and greasier. In addition, our skin is more stressed by regular shaving and therefore more prone to impurities and acne. On the other hand, men's connective and muscle tissues are stronger and better at keeping in moisture. This means that men get wrinkles later on in life—and fewer of them. Unfortunately, men are more at risk for skin cancer than women are. According to a recent study, three times as many men were affected, as their skin contains fewer antioxidants. That's why a good sunscreen and free radical binding grooming products are essential—not just when you're on vacation.

P.S. By the way: many people claim that inexpensive creams are just as good or even better than luxury products. I beg to differ. For sometimes, the more expensive creams are more effective—for example, I feel more well-groomed when using luxury cosmetics than after listlessly spackling my face with some cheap paste or other. The placebo effect is not confined to medicine. As long as you can afford it ...

Detox — Spring Cleaning from the Inside

The path to beauty is not an easy one.

Without a doubt, the most difficult part is getting off your ass and realizing that it's time for a real overhaul! But if your best friends keep telling you, "Man, you're looking really tired/ill/overworked/shitty!" then it's high time you signed up for a beauty crash course.

Blemished or sallow skin, rings and bags under your eyes, a jowly look—in short, once you start looking haggard on a good day, then it's time to take action.

The official explanation for your lousy appearance: Our skin excretes harmful substances that have found their way into our bodies, giving us a grey or sallow complexion. At some point, you've got to pay for all those nights spent crawling through the clubs, the liters of high-proof drinks you've drunk, and the regular visits to your nearest fast food outlet at seven in the morning!

Detox — The Terrible Truth

Before you run off to the drugstore, fork over stacks of cash for crappy cosmetics in order to fruitlessly smear it over your rotting flesh, you should first put yourself through a rigorous spring cleaning. But you can leave the broom and the scrubbing brush where they are, because "detox" means nothing other than "detoxifying"—as in, removing pollutants, dross, and all the other nasty things that have built up in your cells over the years from your system. I recommend taking the detox at the beginning of the new year, after all the unhealthy holidays at the end of the old year. That will give you a fresh start, with more energy.

Detoxing during the week is also a great way to get rid of all the toxic waste that has built up over the weekend, to make yourself fresh and lovely for the next bout. It can also effectively clean out the stress of long caffeine-laden days spent in the office from your ashy and pimply body.

The English professor Sir Colin Berry has a great detox motto: "It's easy to detox; just let your body use the great systems it has evolved over thousands of years to get rid of whatever is harming you."

Sounds Great!

But it's not quite that easy. For our body has a number of great ways of detoxifying itself, but over the course of the years it forgets how to use these tools. So, let's give our bodies a hand in detoxifying!

Beware of Online Detox Methods

If you google "detox," you will stumble over all kinds of crazy and unnecessary products. My favorite being the trashy DVD, *10-Day Detox with Kim Wilde*! Kim Wilde? Holy cow, that flabby little starlet with the enormous pores isn't a recommendation for anything at all—except maybe deep-fried chocolate bars. Even if the reviews promise "Ten days in heaven with Kim," and a certain "Spartak" from New York witters on about her "gorgeous body" and the "unbelievable journey" with her on Amazon, spelling certainly doesn't seem to play much of a role in this journey. I am sure you'll do your body and your mind much more good if you just put on "Kids in America" and rock out in your apartment!

There are also plenty of hilarious tests on the Internet to help you find out whether you are already a compelling case for "detox." Questions such as:

- Do you feel tired and depleted in the mornings?
- Does your food sometimes disagree with you?
- Do you ever have digestive problems?
- Do you easily get out of breath when climbing stairs?
- Are you frequently nervous and irritable?
- Do you often suffer from headaches?
- Are their dark circles under your eyes?

Obviously, anyone living a halfway normal lifestyle will probably answer yes to many of these questions. At the end of these tests, one is often exhorted to buy mysterious foot patches that suck all kinds of toxins through the callouses on your feet, eight hours a day. Or the creepy "Liv52" supplements, those (and I quote) "powerful, all-natural liver detoxifiers and healers."

Excuse Me?

But it's not only DVDs and strange fake wellness products, all kinds of everyday items are marketed as "detox" products. Most of them are of course complete nonsense.

The only thing that really helps your cells get rid of toxins on a molecular level are so-called antioxidants. So when buying detox products, and anything else the cosmetic industry promises, keep your eyes open, ask questions and think for yourself!

Beware of Media Myths

Now is a good time to clear up an old myth about cosmetics: If the commercials promise that their products will penetrate to the deepest layers of your skin, that's a lie. All commercially available cosmetics stay on the surface of the skin. They can do a lot of good there, but if they're going to get rid of real wrinkles, or work inside your body, or fulfill similar promises, these products would have to penetrate as deeply as actual medications. So, beauty products that really do change the deeper structures of the skin and eradicate wrinkles are only available with a doctor's prescription.

But one proper, demonstrably effective method of helping the body flush out toxins is laughter. And so the marketing industry has kind of reached its goal, for who wouldn't laugh at those poor boys spending their last dollar at the corner drugstore, thinking the products they buy there will have the same effect as Botox or Hyaluronan?

But How Does Detoxing Actually Work?

The main thing a detox requires is a lot of discipline, because you will have to totally transform your day-to-day life.

First of all, you should set the period of time you want to "detox" for. Ten days are a good basic period for an intensive detox. Then you need to start dialing back on your daily consumption of toxins. The best way to do this is to buy all your food from an "organic" perspective—so, no artificial aromas, no flavor enhancers, and no preservatives.

Instead of coffee or black tea you'll now be drinking nothing but organic fruit juice and water—lots of water! Your top priority, especially after a long binge, is to take in sufficient fluids. These will flush all the toxins out of your body. Another very good option is a simple chicken broth or a homemade mix of mate-tea, green tea, and lemongrass. This brew is also available commercially under the name Kumsi tea.

All "light" products should be dispensed with. For example, don't replace sugar with some nasty surrogate substance that does your body more harm than good—it may lead your body to believe it's getting some high-fat sustenance while instead causing excessive water retention, which can lead to pretty unhealthy reactions. So, eat light, but only if it's light naturally and not because some scientist has made it "light." Your menu should include lots of fruit and vegetables, especially mangos, which soothe the intestines; strawberries, which have a high vitamin C content (as do the old standby, bell-peppers); avocados; and loads of citrus fruits.

Meat, on the other hand, should be cut out of your diet for the time being, as should most candies and confectionaries, which you shouldn't be eating anyway. Everything in the deep-freeze or a can needs to stay there and not find its way into your stomach.

If you're going to take this really seriously, you'll stop eating altogether. The fashionable term for this is "dinner canceling," which should make abundantly clear what detoxing actually is. The entire business used to be called "fasting," which had a terrible granola-cruncher image. It just goes to show how a clever name change can be great PR ...

The great thing about detoxing is that the smallest adjustment has an almost immediately noticeable effect—sensational bowel movements and considerably more energy.

The Enemy in Your Home

But your food is not the only source of toxins. Your own home can be more toxic than you think. Many a man has furnished his home with killers without realizing it. For example, the pressboard that forms the basis of most cheap shelves contains noxious substances such as formaldehyde, which evaporates over the years and builds up in your cells. So, it's always best to invest in real wood—or at least ask about which substances have gone into the fabrication of the furniture of your choice.

The same goes for the paint and varnish on your walls, carpeting and laminate flooring: All of these need to be completely toxin-free so that they don't slowly-but-surely poison you. So, when choosing paint for your walls, always buy organic, despite the cost, otherwise your walls will breathe chemicals into every room.

These walls or damp corners can swiftly become a breeding ground for fungi that can cause allergies or even cancer. So, make sure there's enough proper ventilation, even if you would prefer your bear-cave to

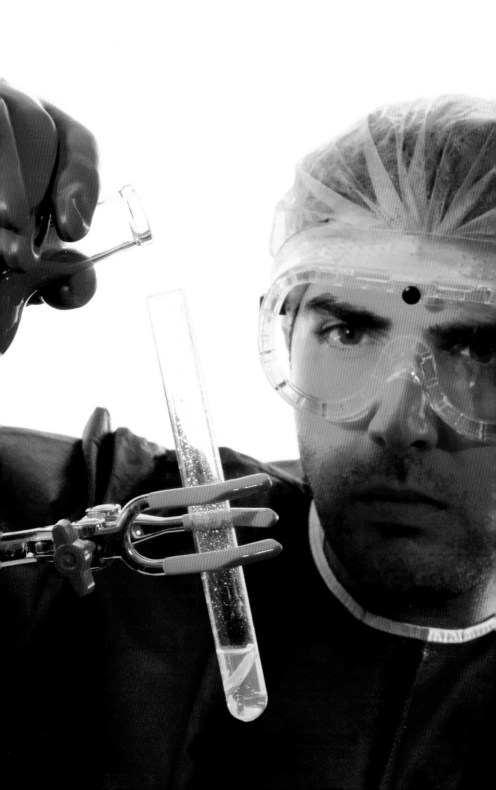

actually smell like one. And for all you golden-shower practitioners: Always make sure that even the darkest corners have a chance to dry out properly after an intense piss-party!

Electrosmog is also highly toxic. This consists of radiation emitted by electronic devices. It has a deleterious effect on your sleep patterns and causes anxiety and even illness. Your bedroom in particular should not contain any electronic devices. So, no bedside TVs, and leave your laptop outside. As most people are already aware, mobile phones have no business anywhere near your sleeping area.

All of these changes will ensure that toxins and pollutants have less chance of building up in our cells. Certain plants, by the way, are great antidotes. Mother Nature will selflessly help you detoxify. So, decorate your apartment with ficus trees, dracaena plants or philodendrons—these are effective toxin-filters.

Fit and Fresh

Of course, proper exercise is an important part of detox. Your low-energy diet will probably prevent you from doing any high-performance sports. But a gentle run in the fresh air is a good start. And if you'd rather join the pensioners in the park, you can clip on your sticks and start Nordic walking. Oxygen and exercise will stimulate your metabolism and speed up the removal of toxins from your blood.

A much better—but sadly, pretty unmanly—option is yoga. You can even find a special form of "detox yoga." This consists of pretty simple exercises that stimulate blood flow to the liver and the metabolic processes there. Your blood is squeezed out of your muscles and internal organs. And you can do all this with exercises such as the "seated forward bend," the "half spinal twist," or the "shoulder-stand," which stimulate the kidneys, the pancreas, the intestines, the liver, and the spleen. The "sun salute," performed every morning, is especially popular—but to be honest, my personal mood during detoxing generally hits rock bottom in the mornings and I don't feel like saluting anyone—not even the sun.

Optimizing

If that's not enough for you, a visit to the sauna will help you sweat out the dross from your cells, and a good massage will stimulate your body's detoxifying systems.

What else? Turning your life over to detox really does have a positive effect, making you feel fresher and more relaxed, so that, following your body's spring-clean, you can start optimizing the rest. So that every man can look as hot as he actually is naturally …

Exfoliating — New Skin, New Me

Once you've cleaned your insides up with a detox, it's time to get matched up on the outside!

There is a point in the life of every man when a look in the mirror tells him it is time to declare war on the aging process!

Parties, stress, cigarettes, and alcohol—all of these will leave their mark, and your jowls will start to hang limply from your face. But it's not just a riotous lifestyle that can make itself felt in pale, blemished skin. Too much sun or cold can also make your skin age faster. All of these factors can make your skin lose its ability to regenerate itself—old cells are no longer released properly to make room for fresh, shiny skin. In addition, those first nasty age freckles start to crop up, and then it's good-bye to your youthful erotic glow. But proper care can do a lot to keep the traces left by day-to-day life in check. But the basis for any real success is getting rid of your old skin—and you can do that with a good exfoliating scrub!

But not all scrubs are the same! There are innumerable products available for every skin type, dermatologists can prescribe medicinal scrubs, and there are plenty of alternatives for DIY fans who prefer to mix their own miracle creams. Deciding on which exfoliating scrub to use depends on your own preferences, the amount of cash you are prepared to spend, and on the type of damage you wish to eliminate.

What Kinds of Exfoliating Scrubs Are There?

The Run-of-the-Mill Scrub

There are exfoliating scrubs available from pretty much every outlet, for every requirement and every price. But first you should have a dermatologist determine your skin type. Then it's off to a good store and time to buy the appropriate goo. Use it according to the instructions and you'll soon be admiring your shiny new reflection in the mirror! Most available facial scrubs generally use fine or slightly coarser abrasive substances or enzymes to remove old cells. You will have to try out a few products to find out which one is right for you. I would personally recommend using very fine abrasive particles in a skin scrub, as in my experience these are a lot more effective than the coarse particles used in many cheaper products. But they are all effective, some more, and some less so. Once you've found the right product for your skin type, you will actually be able to slip down from your real age, say forty years, to an estimated mid-thirty—at least, that is my personal experience.

Professional Peels

If you want to give your face an even more drastic rejuvenation treatment, you're going to need professional help. Beauty clinics and surgeons can supply a number of treatments with varying degrees of strength. In microdermabrasion treatments, the skin is suctioned up by a mechanical nozzle while at the same time fine microcrystals sand off your skin like a sandblaster. That way, old particles of skin are blown away to reveal the fresh skin underneath. This is ideal for people with sallow or tired skin, or large pores. The treatment is painless, your face will be slightly reddened afterwards, but after only a few hours you can go out again, without any obvious traces betraying you.

Other Scrubs

The so-called "business peel" is slightly more intensive. Over the course of several weeks, fine layers of the facial skin are removed with a variety of fluids. This may sound a bit harsh, but it is one of the most unobtrusive exfoliating methods, as this relatively gentle treatment does not leave any traces. The problem is, this procedure takes up a lot of time. The preparation alone can take up to six weeks. On the other hand, the change is less sudden—the rejuvenating process looks more natural. The treatment definitely results in a fresher, smoother look that will stay with you for a long time.

For anyone who doesn't have that much time to spend but would like fast results, there's the "medium peel." This involves aggressive substances burning away the top layer of your skin. This process entails being unable to venture out on the streets for a couple of days, unless you want to be responsible for road accidents and crying children. Because the day after treatment, your skin will begin to tighten, and after two to three days

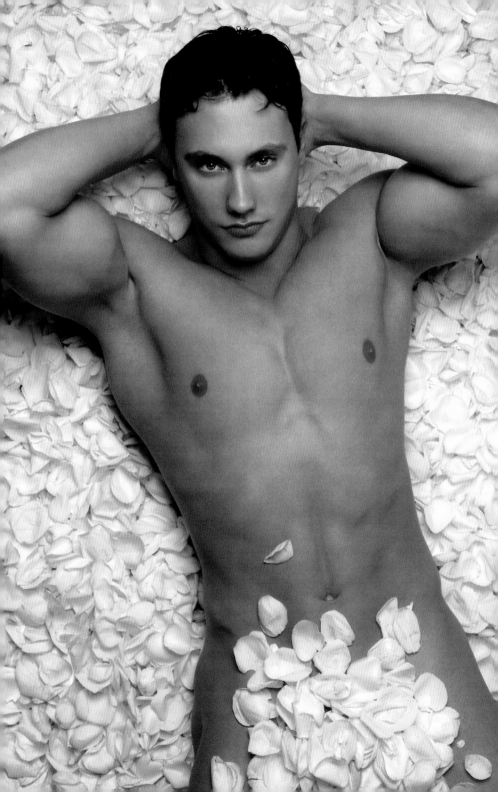

it will darken—and then peel off. The whole thing looks just as gnarly as it sounds. But once you've survived the zombie-phase, you're be as good as new!

If you want to say good-bye entirely to your old self, then a "deep peel" can help—a painful procedure that takes off several layers of the skin on your face right down to the connective tissue. Immediately after treatment, you'll look like something straight out of a horror movie. This procedure is only recommended if you suffer from a serious skin disorder or acute youth obsession. For it will be almost impossible to lead a normal life afterwards. Not only will your skin grow back looking fake and waxy, you will henceforth have to avoid all kinds of sunlight. Whether or not having an unnaturally smooth and tight-skinned face that looks as if your ears were stuck in a vice is worth the price of sitting on the beach covered in a thick layer of cream and an enormous sun hat is up to you.

Do It Yourself

Back to the more agreeable methods of scrubbing the traces of age off your face! I'm actually not a big fan of homemade cosmetics, but I'm willing to make an exception with exfoliating scrubs. These are easy to make, highly effective, generally taste great, and have no chemical additives.

You can easily and effectively mix cane sugar with olive oil to a thick paste. Massage the paste into your skin with circling motions, allow it to take effect briefly before washing it off with lots of warm water and admiring the results.

Another tasty method is to mix honey and curd with lots of sugar and stir till creamy. Apply this to your face, rub it in, and leave it on for a few minutes. The honey and curd will give your skin added moisture and tone. Then wash it all off and enjoy your youthful glow.

The following exotic fruit mask will make your skin smooth and supple: Mash up a banana, add a puréed quarter papaya, and blend with two tablespoons of sugar. Rub in gently, let it sit, and then wash it off again and you'll be glowing like a freshly-plucked fruit.

Create kissable lips with a special lip scrub. For who's going to want to kiss crusty, chapped lips? Just mix up olive oil with some salt to a paste and carefully massage this into your lips until they tingle. Then wipe it off with a soft cloth and apply some moisturizer. Not only is a sleek mouth a lot tastier than a rough one, stimulating circulation to your lips will also make them bigger. But you'll have to rub long and hard before you can compete with the likes of Angelina Jolie.

What's good for the face can't be bad for the rest of your body. Old skin cells should be removed regularly, from neck to toe. That way, you'll look quite a bit younger in your birthday suit as well.

For this, I like to use a coffee-based scrub supposedly used by prickly Naomi Campbell. First, rub oil onto your entire body. Then make a paste out of granulated coffee or five table-spoons of freshly brewed ground coffee and rub it into your skin. Rinse well with water! This will deep-cleanse and rejuvenate your skin, leaving you pink and gleaming like a little piglet. But the best part is, caf-feine will also stimulate your body's fat-burning processes. A scrub that makes you slim *and* beautiful—what more could you ask for?

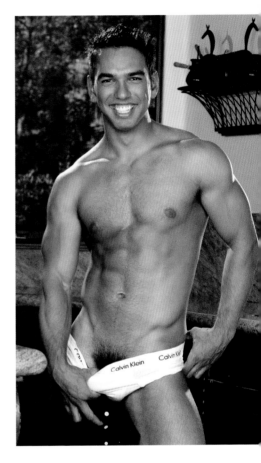

How Much Grooming Does a Man Need?

I think we can all agree that a daily grooming routine is now obligatory for men as well. Which is why I won't go into too much detail about the stuff that should be a given. But as a checklist for your daily grooming routine, here's my bathroom top ten:

10 Toothpaste and a toothbrush! This should really be a given, but frighteningly enough, one man in seven will dispense with brushing his teeth every night. And one in five will regularly skip brushing every morning. Yuck!

TOP TEN BATHROOM CHECKLIST

9 A mild, neutral pH-value wash lotion to gently cleanse your face on a regular basis. A lipid-balancing shower or bath gel is of course equally important, to make sure the rest of your body is beautifully and thoroughly clean.

8 Deodorant! OK, I know there is a large faction within the gay community that's into sweat. But please, keep it to yourselves. Among complete strangers during day to day life, the way some guys let their armpits emanate all kinds of fumes borders on olfactory assault. I don't want to have to smell you and neither do many, many others. After all, you can always get an unscented deodorant!

7 A good moisturizer for everyday use on your face is also indispensable. This will supply your skin with everything it needs to remain taut for as long as possible. You should definitely choose a moisturizer with UV protection filters, because few things makes your skin age as quickly as too much unprotected exposure to sunlight. If you want to treat yourself, choose a product that also contains an anti-aging complex.

6 Naturally, a good eye cream should also be part of your daily routine. Why? You'll find out in the relevant chapter!

5 To keep not just the skin on your face nice and supple, you should regularly use a body lotion after showering or bathing. For best effects, apply to your skin while it's still damp.

4 A well-groomed man should definitely have all the necessary utensils for nail care in his bathroom. See the relevant chapter for details.

3 A blemish concealer stick is an indispensable part of every good household. It should cover blemishes with a natural color, without getting dry and flaky, and should definitely act as a disinfectant on the inflamed area.

2 Every man should have a really good shaving kit. This includes a non-irritant shaving gel, a non-alcohol based and unscented aftershave, and a good razor—the more blades, the better.

1 As a final touch, a well-groomed man should have a good cologne with a fragrance that suits him. I'll explain how to find the right fragrance in detail in a later chapter.

Bald Is Beautiful

Fashions come and go, but a bald head will always be sexy! I've personally been wearing the "skin-cap" since I was sixteen and that's made me absolutely down with the latest trend at least five times, but has also placed me beyond the pale of fashion about five times as well. By now, there aren't really any other hairstyling alternatives left for me, as my head would only sprout a rudimentary fringe of hair anyway. So, I just sit back and let the current wave of hair fashion pass me by and wait until my look is back in style. I actually don't care what style is currently in fashion, I think a bald head is always hot—as do many other guys. It's as soft as a baby's bottom and guaranteed to catch the eye, inviting

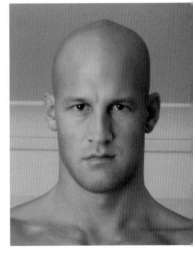

nice boys to stroke it and bad boys to think dirty thoughts about it. A bald head will turn even the more mature gentlemen out there into a universal sex symbol. Examples: Bruce Willis and Vin Diesel! Imagine either of them with hair! No way! The sight of these men's thinning heads of hair might arouse pity, but certainly not an erection. Baldness is the most sincere of hairstyles: it gives you an unimpeded, undistorted view of the guy's face—with no cunning styling, no trendy frills to distract from a dull and ugly mug.

Apart from that, going bald saves you undreamt-of amounts of time. Get out of bed, wipe it off, and you're ready to go. No more washing, blow-drying, or styling—precious hours of your life restored to you!

So, off with that unnecessary fluff on your head!

How to Shave Your Head

Pick the right time to shave your head. That means you should never break out the razor during the evenings or after a meal, as those are the times when the risk of injury is the greatest. This is because the blood supply to the vessels lying directly below the skin is greater at those times than at others. The best time would be in the morning before breakfast. Or as foreplay for a prolonged sex session, because you shouldn't do that on a full stomach either.

You should also wait till after shaving before you take a shower, because otherwise your scalp will swell up and part of the follicles will be "swallowed." You won't get a clean shave that way.

If you take a sharp razor to your long hair, you'll be setting yourself up for a bloody endeavor. So, once you've decided on the ideal time, cut your hair as short as possible with clippers. That will also give you a last opportunity to take stock of the situation in the mirror and to decide whether you really want to shave it all off—the "last exit" for baldy newcomers, so to speak.

Now it's time to get serious! You'll need high-quality shaving cream. Do not use any of the cheapo products, as these are generally too abrasive for your sensitive scalp. Choose the gentlest cream you can find—if possible, one that contains aloe vera. That way, shaving your head will still be slippery fun, even for a beginner.

Now apply the shaving cream evenly and let it sit there for a few minutes. This will allow the hairs to stand up, making them easier to chop off. Then shave your hair with the grain, otherwise you may easily just nick the hairs without removing them completely—just as when you're shaving your beard. Pulling your scalp taught against the shave will make it extremely smooth and it will be easier to remove the hairs in less accessible places. It also reduces the risk of cutting yourself. It's better to feel your way through the shave, as you can't always check yourself in the mirror while shaving your head—so take your time, take care, and relax.

It is very important that you use the right razor. Cheap razors are a nightmare for any scalp, as they are often awkward and not sharp enough. So, stay clear of disposable razors!

You'll need the best razor for the best shaved head! This means that the razor should have as many blades as possible and should ideally be unused—after all, the blades get blunter with every use and will start to pull at your scalp rather than cutting properly. You can also buy special razors, such as the "headblade," which looks like a small snowmobile and is constructed so that the blade is always at the right angle to the head, while the bent handle gives you a better grip. However, this tool takes a little practice before you can smoothly scythe away the stubble.

There is no real alternative to shaving with a razor. Applying hair removal creams—such as the ones the girls use on their legs—to your scalp is generally not a good idea. For this mostly leads to the "Chernobyl-Survivor" look—a few pathetic tufts of hair struggling for survival on top of your bright scarlet head. There are some gentler exceptions, such as the Indian natural depilation method that uses only sugar, citric acid, water, and sunflower oil. But ultimately, you should always stay on the safe side and use a sharp five-blader.

Once your scalp is smooth and strokably soft after shaving, it will need special care. Now please don't pour aftershave over it—your screams of pain might panic the neighbors. The ingredients in regular aftershave are far too abrasive for your scalp. Instead, I recommend using a gentle lotion or a cooling gel—with no added alcohol or fragrances, of course. This will soothe and protect your scalp and make your dome gleam like a billiard ball.

In conclusion, all you can do now is hope that everyone else thinks your new head-style is as hot as you do.

By the way: There's a shaving solution for scaredy cats. If you're undecided as to whether or not to chop the hair off your head, I suggest you go visit your nearest makeup artist's supply store. They will have rubber baldy wigs that, with a little practice and makeup, can turn any hippy into a true blue skinhead. These things won't survive a wild night at the disco or a vigorous hookup of course, they are far too delicate for that. But they're good enough if you just want to test people's reactions to your new look. And yes, your head will itch horribly—but if you're such a coward, you deserve to suffer!

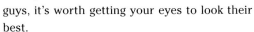

Eye-Catching Eyes

Goldie Hawn uses hemorrhoid cream to get rid of the bags under her eyes, Cindy Crawford sticks raw potato slices on her eyes, and my friend Shirley puts her eighteen-month-old son's ice-cold teething-rings on her tired eyes. Everyone knows of some way of getting your eyes into better shape. And as you generally use them to make first contact with hot

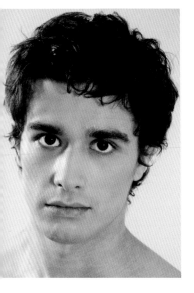

guys, it's worth getting your eyes to look their best.

Lovely eyes are however not just a matter of good grooming. Your eyesight should also be the apple of your eye. Because nearsighted people tend to squint imperceptibly, creating deep crows-feet and nasty frown wrinkles between the eyebrows.

If nature has endowed you with blue eyes, you will be perceived as not only more attractive by people around you, but also as more intelligent—this has been scientifically proven. However, I have also had days in which a pair of red and swollen baboon's butts stared back at me from my eye sockets. Here are a few effective tips on how to turn your watery eyes back into sparkling sex-magnets:

Proper Eye Care

You might think "I just rub a plain moisturizer around my eyes, that should do it!"—and you would be wrong! The delicate skin around your eyes is only 0.5 millimeters thick, four times as fine as the rest of the skin on your face. That makes it more prone to wrinkles and especially sensitive to greasy creams. As soon as you hit your twenties, the first signs of age will start to dig in around your eyes, and only an expensive face-lift can eliminate them. So it's definitely worth starting proper eye care early on.

A good eye cream should be part of every well-groomed gentleman's routine. However, do make sure that you are not over-sensitive or allergic to any of the ingredients.

But what's even more important than the effect the product has is the way you apply it: If you smear and rub it in around your eyes, you will achieve the opposite of the desired effect. Your skin is too delicate to survive this ordeal without creating wrinkles. Always apply eye cream with your—relatively weak—ring finger. Use the cream under and around the eye. Never apply it directly to the lid, otherwise the stuff will be carried—in the blink of an eye—into the eye itself, which won't feel great. After applying it with your ring finger, tap lightly over the cream until it is completely absorbed. This will also stimulate the blood circulation and the removal of waste products from your skin. But good grooming is not enough to maintain good-looking eyes. Good care also means good nutrition! To keep your eagle eyes keen and focused and to avoid having to scrunch them up, you need to be taking in enough of the right vitamins: vitamin A, vitamin C, and vitamin E. Retinol and beta-carotene are also essential for good vision, as these are both raw materials for visual purple, which is necessary for the proper functioning of the light receptors in your retina. To ensure that you get enough of these essential substances, eat sufficient quantities of the following tasty snacks: parsley, bell peppers, broccoli, white cabbage, kiwis, and citrus fruits. Carrots, apricots, beetroot, papaya and lettuce, nuts, asparagus, and kale. Drinking a glass of tomato juice daily is also great—and not just for your eyes!

To avoid straining your eyes, causing them to age more rapidly, avoid the following:

- getting cigarette smoke in your eyes
- staring at your computer screen for too long
- letting the air in your home get too dry
- overheating the air in your home
- not getting enough sleep
- too much sun

Speaking of the sun, to keep your eyes looking youthful, you will absolutely need high-quality sunglasses in the summer. Choose a pair with the highest UV protection rating and wide frames to block out sunlight from the sides.

Pretty much everyone is familiar with this effect: swollen and bloated eyes after a long night. This is caused by a build-up of lymphatic fluids that haven't drained quickly enough. Cold cucumber slices laid on the eyes really do help. Another effective solution is to brew up a bag of black tea, stick it in the freezer and then lay it on your closed eyes for fifteen minutes.

If you constantly suffer from swollen eyes, you might want to try changing your diet! Less salt, less caffeine, and less alcohol!

By the way, dark circles under the eyes are not always caused by sleep deprivation. They can also be hereditary or caused by disease—if the problem persists, it's best to consult your doctor. There's no effective cream for these dark circles, so try using a special concealer.

And What About My Eyebrows?

Gorgeous eyes need a suitable frame—your eyebrows! Sadly, more and more young guys choose to go for hysterically plucked eyebrows, like those of some ghetto-type stylist. Why? Those thinly plucked eyebrows with their feminine slant make the hottest guy look like a drag queen who's forgotten to take off his makeup. Men should have men's eyebrows and these have a totally different shape than women's eyebrows: they aren't wildly arched and thin, as if they'd been drawn on with a Sharpie. A well-kempt man's eyebrow still retains its natural shape, it's just the hairs that are too long and stick out that need removing! This is quite easy to do: Dampen a toothbrush, brush your eyebrow hairs down, and cut off anything that's too long. Then pluck out any hairs that stand out and are obviously in the wrong place. And there you are: well-groomed eyebrows!

You should always check yourself in the mirror while grooming. Because a couple of wrongly plucked hairs are enough to make your eyebrow look as if it's suffering from avian flu. There should be no hair at all between your eyebrows above your nose, otherwise your face will look angry. So, go to town there!

Here's a tip for all you vain boys out there from dear old Marlene Dietrich. Before going out, draw a line on the inside of your lower lid with a white or light blue eyeliner. This will open your eye up and make them look magic—giving you an enchanting gaze.

Accentuating your eyelashes can be tricky but very effective. Just a touch of color there will give your gaze a new, brighter intensity. I strongly discourage dyeing them yourself, though. This should be left to a trained stylist. Because unless you get the color and tone exactly right, you'll end up looking like a randy panda. The dye should look subtle, the effect will be best that way. After the dyeing procedure with your stylist, you will need to take a good shower, as there will be lot of dye residue left in your eyelashes, which can be easily washed out with water. Then you can mingle with other people in public again and start catching a few hot looks.

What Else Can I Do for My Eyes?
Here are a few simple and effective exercises for everyone who regularly puts their eyes under a lot of strain, for instance by staring at a computer screen for hours on end. These exercises will not only strengthen your vision, but also the muscles around your eyes, which will help prevent wrinkles.

Exercising Your Eyes
Yawning can help! Hard to believe, but a good yawn will tense and relax all the muscles in your face, as well as those in the back of your neck and your back. Taking a deep breath gives your brain a hearty extra dose of oxygen and stimulates tear production. This will keep your eyes moist for those yearning gazes.

"Refocusing" is a recognized training principle. This means tensing the eye muscles in near focus and then relaxing them in far focus. To do this, focus on an object about twelve inches from your face. Keep your gaze there for a moment, then look into the distance—for example, out of the window. Then focus back on the object, and then into the distance again. Repeat ten times, and you've got yourself a great workout for your eye muscles.

The next exercise sounds ridiculously easy but it's very effective. Just close your eyes and try to relax them. Stay like this for several minutes. This simple exercise protects the eye from the light and lets the inner eye muscles relax properly. But this exercise is also good for the external eye muscles, as the eyes move apart and upwards slightly when relaxed, which allows these muscles to relax as much as possible.

Look at something green! I'm not kidding—looking at a green surface relaxes the eye most of all. This is also one reason why blackboards used to be green. Because that particular shade of green proved to be best for tireless vision.

The following massage technique is an incredibly effective relaxation exercise. Gently squeeze the bridge of your nose with your thumb and middle finger, while your index finger presses down on the region between your eyebrows. Then make circling motions with all three fingers, applying gentle pressure. Repeated several times a day for just thirty seconds, this exercise will relax all the muscles around your eyes and prevent crow's feet from forming.

The last technique is the most strenuous. It's important to stay relaxed and to repeat each exercise eight times.

Start off by focusing your gaze to the far right, without moving your head. Then quickly move your eyes as far to the left as you can go—and then back again. Back and forth.

Do the same with your gaze, going up and down, top right to bottom left, and top left to bottom right—repeating each exercise eight times. Finish by lowering your gaze and rolling your eyes around in wide circles.

All these exercises are the same as any kind of sport—the more you train, the more effective they are. But don't let anyone catch you at it. For admittedly, they do make you look like a complete weirdo, or someone caught in the throes of a really bad LSD trip.

Dat Ass!

What's the second thing a man's lovely eyes will focus on? Correct: dat ass!

A clean-shaven head is hot enough, but shaved junk has its advantages too, as it saves you from laboriously picking someone else's pubes out of your mouth after a blow job. But some gay boys are just as fond of a smoothly shaved butt.

Whether you licking, fucking, or just looking—gorgeous! Although fans of thick natural growth in the genital area are on the rise, the overwhelming majority would rather stick their tongues in between two smooth cheeks and not into a matted jungle—it's just a question of taste. (If you'll pardon the cheap pun ...)

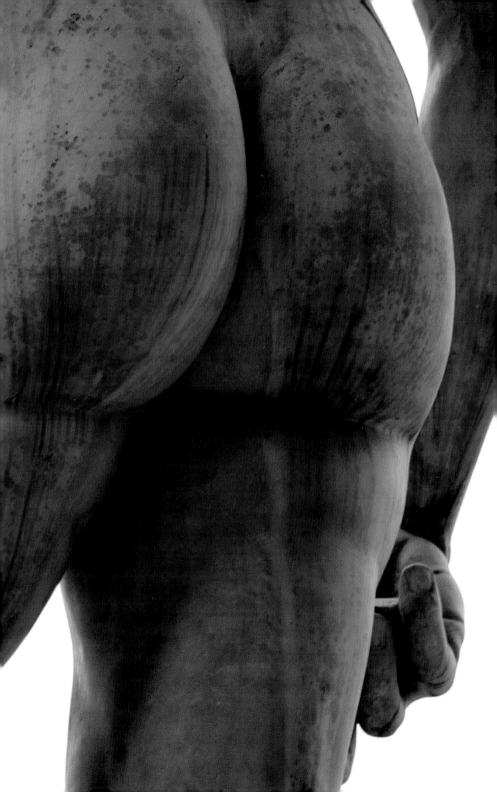

To get your firm butt setting men's pulses racing, here is my plan for shaving your ass, turning your bearded moon into two enticing fleshy hummocks:

SHAVING YOUR ASS

1 Fill up a large bowl with warm water and place it strategically in the shower or the bathtub. Make sure you have enough light!

2 Conveniently place a very good, very sharp razor with lots of blades nearby, and next to it, a hand-mirror and shaving gel for sensitive skin. Avoid shaving cream as this will obstruct your view of the object of your shave. Steer clear of disposable razors. These should not be used on your sensitive behind and will only cause unpleasant cuts.

3 Strip off!

4 Moisten your butt with lots of warm water and massage the shaving gel into the skin and hair on your behind, getting your short-and-curlies nice and soft.

5 Warm up the razor thoroughly with warm water. Then start shaving along the curve of your cheek from bottom to top. Don't be too hesitant, otherwise you may cut yourself. Employ short, confident strokes using your entire arm and not just the wrist—that will make for a cleaner shave.

6 Rinse off the razor after every stroke to prevent it from becoming clogged with hair.

7 Carefully work your way from the outside inwards and keep checking your progress in the hand mirror.

8 Be especially careful in the very sensitive region around your anus. The skin is extremely delicate there and easily injured. Now aren't you glad you made sure you had enough light in your bathroom? Because checking out the dark depths of your ass crack is no easy task.

9 Once the last tiny hair is gone and your butt is soft as a baby's, you've made it. Now disinfect it with an appropriate product to reduce the risk of ingrown hairs, otherwise you'll break out in pimples. But don't use anything that contains alcohol, otherwise people in your street will think you're slaughtering a pig. It really is that painful!

10 Present your smooth butt to as many admiring gazes as you can—after all, it has to be worth the effort! As with your beard, your sleek behind will stay hairless for varying lengths of time. If you've got record-breaking stubble, your super soft glory may be over within twelve hours' time. There are very few fans of the unpleasant scratching sensation caused by the hair growing back. But if you're lucky, your behind will stay perfect for weeks, until it starts growing a soft layer of bum fluff.

Hands — Sticky Fingers

This really cheap, totally gay segue takes us from sexy asses to hands to match!

Straight women and gay men have quite a few fantasies in common that are completely foreign to straight men. Or are there many straight men dreaming of a busty blonde with nasty calloused hands? No, the girls need to be soft and gentle! On the other hand, there are pitiable women and silly gay men who think they will find sexual fulfillment if a rough Mediterranean fisherman grabs them with his horny hands and "takes" them in a fit of unbridled passion. Yeah, I'd like to see that. I wonder how they'd react to some guy stinking of fish lying in bed and tearing holes in the high thread-count bedclothes with his calloused fingers. "Salt on Our Skin?" More like "Wire Brush on My Dick!"

In real life, a man with well-cared-for hands is much more popular and successful. From the job interview to the first date—the impression your hands give are often the deciding factor between your enterprise's success or failure.

The "rough hand" problem is familiar not only to hard-working fishermen, but also to pretty much every fitness freak. The gyms are packed with boys with big muscles—and even bigger callouses on their cracked hands. Daily barbell training will make your body beautiful, but it will also give you ugly lumps between your fingers—and unfortunately it is those details that make a man attractive. Or not.

Sometimes rough hands can point to disorders of the skin. The possible causes can range from stress to hormonal imbalances. So, if your hands just won't get any softer, in spite of excellent care, have a doctor check them out. Otherwise, it's the same as ever: The sooner you start your care routine, the longer the benefit when you get older!

How to Have Nice Hands

The skin on your hands is especially thin and has no subdermal layer of fat. So, there's not much standing between environmental wear and tear or abrasive cleaning detergents and your skin's protective barrier. Your skin will lose its moisture quickly, making it cracked and dry. Germs and other harmful substances can then find their way into your body through these fine cracks in your skin—and as you can probably imagine, that's not healthy.

Excessive movement of the joints also put constant strain on the skin—so the floppy wrist brigade had better not come crying to me if they get really wrinkly hands early on.

Proper Care of Your Hands

1. Wash your hands—including your nails—properly several times a day with a mild, neutral pH-value soap. This will not only get them clean, it is also the best way to protect yourself from viral infections such as swine flu. Most viruses and bacteria enter the body via the hands and the mucous membranes—i.e., via your eyes, nose, or mouth when you touch them with your fingers. If your hands are especially calloused, rub them down well with pumice stone several times a day. This should quickly remove the traces of years of lifting weights.

2. After washing, apply a specialized, non-greasy cream to your hands. Depending on your age, your daily care product should contain pre- or anti-aging substances, vitamins, and UV protection. If you've already got age freckles or pigmentation on your skin, a skin lightening product can help.

   There are a lot of good products on the market now that will subtly bleach the affected areas without putting too much strain on the skin.

3. During the nighttime, give your hands a rest and let them regenerate. I don't mean you have to forgo your evening masturbation session. Try pampering your paws with a special night cream. To increase effectiveness, wear a pair of cotton gloves over your moisturized hands overnight—you'll have amazingly soft hands the next morning. Obviously, you should only do this if you're planning on spending the night alone in bed. Very few things are less erotic than spending the night lying next to a snoring guy in greasy cotton gloves.

4. Once a week you should treat your hands to an exfoliating scrub, the same as your face. This will remove dead cells and stimulate the circulation—your fingers will have a new shine to them. Apply an intensive moisturizer afterwards, as this will penetrate more deeply into your skin after exfoliating. You can find all kinds of effective products in specialist stores, from luxury ampoules with highly concentrated serums to hand masks.

5. Pamper your hands with a paraffin bath, a luxury spa treatment for rough hands. You can have this done by a beautician or invest in a cost-effective appliance for home use. There are a number of procedures for paraffin baths, but this one is the safest: After exfoliating, your hands are coated with a concentrated hand care mask, covered with plastic gloves, and then placed in warm liquid paraffin. This will make your skin perspire, opening the pores so that the active substances can penetrate into your cells, improving circulation while retaining the moisture on your skin. It's like a hand sauna. After the wax hardens, you can just pull it off with the gloves. The combined warmth and moisturizer will make your hands incredibly soft and, speaking from my own experience, I can only say that even the toughest guy will enjoy being pampered with hands like that. Soft hands don't make you a softy.

    If you don't want to get too elaborate, you can give your hands a twenty-minute bath in warm olive oil once a week, this will also yield fantastic results. By the way, you can do the same for your feet. They are often even more in need of a proper pampering.

    My grandma always had hands as soft as a baby's because she bathed them regularly in a mixture of warm buttermilk and chamomile tea for twenty minutes.

How to Care for Your Nails

Hands are not only made of skin. The appearance of your nails is one of the most important indicators of how well-groomed a man is. If the nails don't look right, this will even throw a negative light on your character. That is why you should never have chewed, dirty, or split fingernails! As guys, we don't have the option of hiding our unsightly, blemished nails underneath pretty, artificial stick-ons, the way girls do.

1. The use of chemicals, whether you're house-cleaning or disinfecting your sex toys, can damage your nails just the same as your skin. Soap and water can also make your nails, which consist of horn, brittle and porous. So, when moisturizing your hands, make sure to pay special attention to your nails.

2. Fingernails are a commonly recognized indicator for overall health. Even if you're not completely familiar with the signs, you will unconsciously pick up this information—and quickly decide whether or not you like a person, based on what their nails tell you. Strong, smooth nails, with no ridges or blemishes are a sign of a healthy, fit body. Split, deformed, or dull nails can be a sign of a vitamin or mineral deficiency. Other causes may be allergies, digestive disorders or poor circulation. Yellow nails can be caused by nicotine deposits in heavy smokers, but may also be a sign of a fungus infection—neither of these is very nice.

   So, here's a tip for you smokers: Mix some icing sugar with lemon juice to a paste, apply this to your nails, and wash it off after a few minutes—your smoker's fingers will be pure as the driven snow once again.

3. How long should a man's nails be? Your nails actually serve as a natural protection for your fingertips, so they shouldn't be too short. But as gay men do occasionally stick their hands up each other's butts, their nails short be kept as short as possible to avoid injuring the sensitive tissue around the anus. But that is easier said than done. If you have neither the time nor the patience to practice properly and if you can afford it, you should have a manicure done regularly. There's a manicure studio on pretty much every street corner. When choosing a studio, keep the following in mind: only go to a manicure studio where they use hand files. If any of the ladies working there try to treat your fingers with any kind of electric appliance, get the hell out of there. For a really good manicure can only be accomplished with a hand file. Anything electric will grind off too much, too quickly, and end up destroying your nails.

4. To care for your nails at home, you will need a couple of utensils. Beginners in particular should really make sure to get good quality products. Otherwise your nail will be worn away much faster than you'd like. So, before you start experimenting on yourself, go out and buy the following:

- a good, strong pair of nail scissors
- a four-way nail buffer
- one coarse and one fine nail file

The thinner and weaker your nails are, the finer the grain on your file should be. If you want to be particular, get yourself a cuticle pen as well. I do not recommend using the classic nail clippers as theses will make the edges of your nails brittle.

5. Obviously, the surface of your nails should always be clean. If they are very dirty, go ahead and take a nail brush and some washing detergent to them. Heavy staining, e.g. from nicotine can be removed with the cleaning edge of a nail buffer. Rub the soft gritty surface over the entire surface of your nails, applying light pressure, and they'll be spick-and-span again.

6. Now it's time to shorten them. The best time to attack your nails is after showering or bathing as this will make them nice and soft. Use a stainless pair of scissors to cut your nails to a consistent length, meaning: your nails should never protrude past your fingertips. In contrast to women's nails, a man's nails should never taper off but rather have a square tip and oval sides—it does take a little practice to get your nails perfect. Once you've finished with the scissors, pick up your coarse file and use it to roughly shape your nails. Then use the finer file, which removes much less of your nail, to fine-tune the shape. If you want to be particular, you can use a ceramic file to seal the edge of your nail. This will protect it from splitting and tearing.

7. Cuticles are a special problem for men, as they grow thicker and more quickly than women's do. Important: No matter how horrible your cuticles look, never cut them off! Otherwise they will only grow back more thickly. Use a cuticle pen to apply a fluid to make your cuticles soft and supple so that you can gently, without too much force, push them back with the soft tip. Rub off any small shreds that are left with a soft cloth. This will give you a great, well-groomed appearance.

8. Finish off by buffing your nails—just like you would a good car. Use the buffer side of your four-way buffer to smooth off those ridges. If you really want your nails to shine, get yourself a buffing kit with a leather buffer and powder. You sprinkle the powder over your nails and rub it hard with the buffer until it's gone—this will give your nails

a long lasting high gloss. Transparent nail polish is becoming more common among men, and it will keep your nails shining for weeks. Visually, however, it is a little bold and should only be used if the rest of your body is also styled to an almost unearthly degree of perfection.

Injectable Beauty — The Botox Myth

We could hardly finish off a chapter on good looks without mentioning one of the most frequently debated products of our time—Botox!

We all know by now: Life is easier if you look good. Which is why many people, especially gay men, are prepared to do anything for their looks, even if only to feel and look more attractive to themselves. Whenever the obsession with eternal youth is under discussion, the talk quickly turns to Jocelyn "Catwoman" Wildenstein and Mickey Rourke's wreck of a face. Every newspaper, every radio station, every idiot with something to say will then give voice to cries of, "They've had too much Botox! It's the devil's poison!" That pisses me off to no end!

For Botox would have to be a pretty sensational invention to be responsible for all the deformed faces of those pitiful celebrities. Faces pulled taut, narrow noses, thick lips, high cheekbones, and the transformation of an average-looking American woman into a terrifying catlike creature—and Botox did all of this?

Nonsense!

The duty of the media should actually be to educate the public. But Botox seems to cause a system failure in the cleverest minds behind the editors' desks. There are so many rumors and so much misinformation flying about that I feel it is my duty as a lifestyle writer to try and set the record straight. After all, everyone should be able to decide for himself which methods to consider when wishing to fine-tune his appearance.

First off: Personally, I do not believe anyone should use Botox. Good care is important, but you should really allow yourself to age the way nature intended. After all, every face tells the story of a life and that's what makes it interesting. But of course, I can understand why a guy might want to get himself treated! The best example I know is Matthew, thirty-nine years old, successful in his career, happily in love, and a staunch Botox user. However, you'd never know he used the stuff. I'd never have realized it myself. Matthew simply looks like a well-rested, well-cared-for man—a dashing kind of guy.

It was only after a while that I find out that without Botox, he would have had deep bulldog wrinkles on his forehead, nasty crows-feet around his eyes, and engrained frown lines above his nose. But thanks to Botox, none of this is to be seen, and he believes that this is the secret to his success.

So, there are worlds lying between what Botox can do when used reasonably and the horrifying pictures you see in the tabloids. To give everyone the opportunity to form his own judgment about the Botox myth, here are the most important facts:

The Truth About Botox

First of all, "Botox" is not the active ingredient, it is merely the name of the product. The same way "Kleenex" is only one of many brands of paper tissues. The stuff has been around for over twenty years and has been documented in thousands of medical studies. If you want to know more, there is plenty for you to look up.

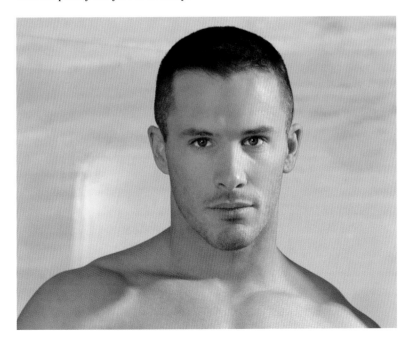

The Botox Myth 1

The Myth: But it's ptomaine poison / a neurotoxin!

Answer: As I've said, "Botox" is just the brand name. The active substance is "Botulinum toxin," a protein which can, of course, occur anywhere on Earth. It is a by-product of decomposing meat or sausage, among others.

The Botox Myth 2

The Myth: Toxin? So, it must be poisonous!

THE BOTOX MYTH

Answer: That depends on the amount. Just as with nearly everything else, the wrong dosage can be fatal. Nobody can ingest a kilo of salt, a hundred aspirin pills, or have nutmeg injected into his veins and live to tell the tale. Is anyone getting upset over salt, aspirin, or nutmeg? No! Nobody would dream of demonizing these things. It's much more important to realize that some of our most effective medications, for example, are based on snake venom.

The Botox Myth 3

The Myth: After treatment your face will look like a death mask!

Answer: That's not entirely false. Again, it depends on the dose. In America, there is a phenomenon called "Frozen Faces," where people who have had too much of the stuff injected into themselves do, in fact, lose all ability to form facial expressions and their faces look like wax masks. But that's the fault of their doctors.

The Botox Myth 4

The Myth: Botox is dangerous!

Answer: We can spare ourselves the answer to that by simply looking at the following comparison: An average treatment means injecting about fifty units into your face. Botox is also used under another name as a medication to help children suffering from spastic equinus foot or cerebral palsy. These children are injected with up to 600 units so that they can walk again. Children whose lives have been so significantly improved by this product would probably be surprised at how dismissively people talk about it.

The Botox Myth 5

The Myth: Botox kills off nerves—you will never be able to feel anything again!

Answer: This is true in part. Botox blocks the transmission of stimuli to the nerves. But as the nervous plexus regenerates all the time, new neural pathways will have grown to transmit the stimuli after about six months. But that also means you will lose the visual effect. You will look just the same as before.

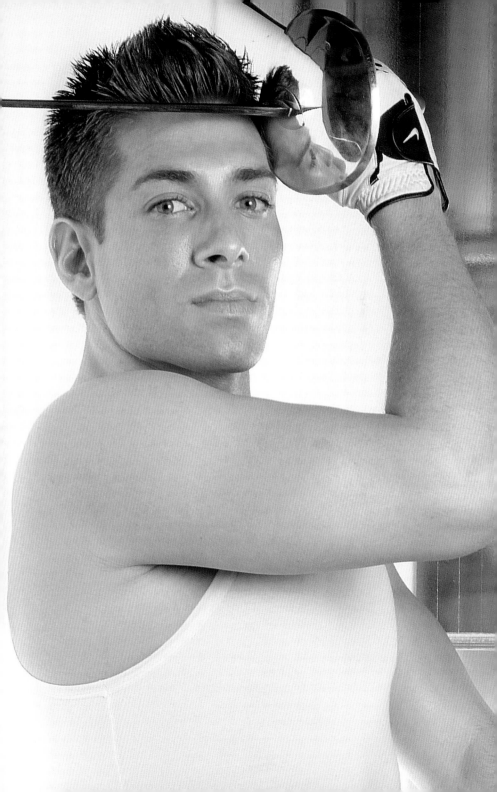

The Botox Myth 6

The Myth: You don't need a needle, you can get organic Botox from the pharmacy!

Answer: This is fraud, pure and simple. Botox is a medication, its use is restricted to certified doctors, and it is not available on the free market. After all, it has to go deep under your skin to be effective. As we have already mentioned, no freely available product can penetrate that deeply (despite what the advertisers would have you believe), and anything else is just a cunningly marketed cosmetic product and will never have the same effect.

The Botox Myth 7

The Myth: Botox hurts!

Answer: Apparently not. The needles used to inject it are very thin so you won't feel anything. There's just the crackle of the needle penetrating the thick layers of skin. You don't feel the substance itself at all. If you do feel pain, that's probably because your doctor can't use his needle properly.

The Botox Myth 8

The Myth: Nothing is known about the long-term effects!

Answer: As I've said before, Botox has been researched for twenty years now. There is hardly another form of medication as well documented. According to the current state of research, there are no long-term effects!

The Botox Myth 9

The Myth: Botox will destroy your face, make your lips swell up, etc.!

Answer: How is it supposed to do that? Those much-desired full lips are achieved by injecting Hyaluronan, for example. Botox isn't used to fill anything up, which is why it can't be used to eliminate deep labial folds (the ones around your mouth) either. In addition, the effects of Botox will subside after a while. Anything that might have been messed up will soon revert back to its original state.

The Botox Myth 10

The Myth: Botox is only for the super rich!

Answer: It depends on your priorities. A good facial treatment can cost up to $400. So, it's definitely not cheap.

The Botox Myth 11

The Myth: Botox will make you lose the ability to form facial expressions!

Answer: This is partly true. Your facial expressions will be inhibited. For example, you won't be able to look angry anymore. Because the muscles responsible have to be incapacitated in order to give you that relaxed, rested expression. But you could see that as a benefit.

That should have cleared up a few of the most common prejudices. Everyone should decide for themselves whether this is a treatment for you or not. Personally, I prefer to take the path of good grooming and mindful living. Above all, I don't for the life of me want anything squirted in my face—at least not Botox.

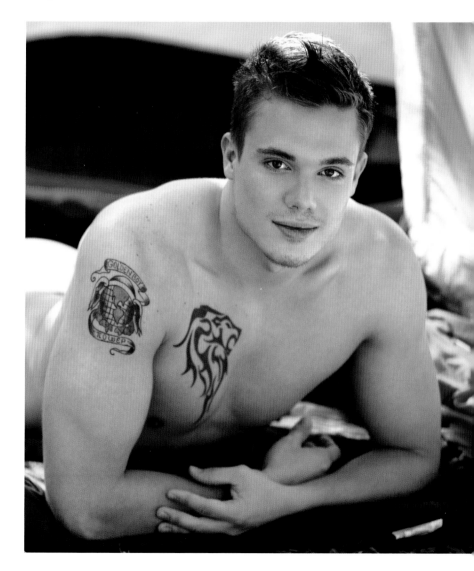

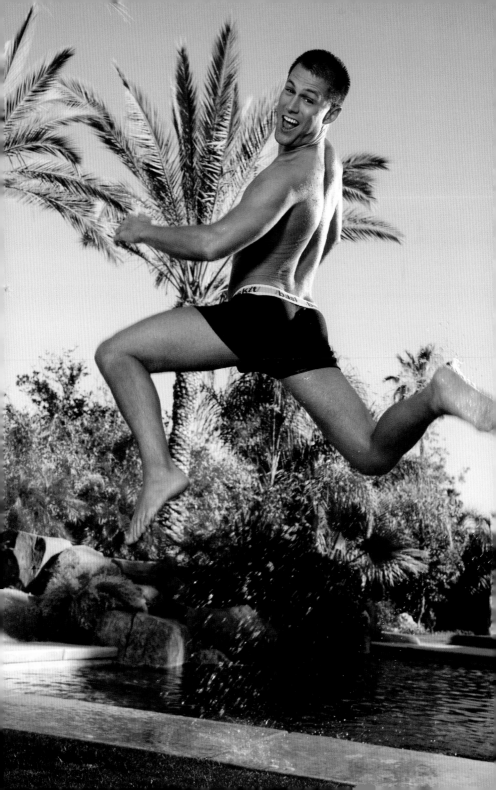

Facts of Life

More practical knowledge to keep any party and any conversation running smoothly.

Breakfast of Champions
The diet industry markets corn flakes to us as the ideal breakfast food. You can't really go wrong there, as the stuff doesn't contain anything at all. You'll find more nutrients in the packaging than you will in the corn flakes.

Cheers!
So, that's why the girls on *Sex and the City* drink so many of those strong Cosmopolitans. The word "Manhattan" was originally an old Indian word meaning "the place we were drunk in".

Bugs
Carmine, the red dye formerly used in Campari, is revoltingly made out of ground up cochineal insects that inhabit the Canary Islands. This dye can be found in all kinds of products, among them, lipstick.

Oh, Right...
Politicians do not lie as much as you would think. Most of them simply rely on the public's ignorance instead. So if politicians talk about a quantum leap, they don't actually mean a fundamental change, but rather that everything will stay the same. A quantum leap is the smallest possible change within a physical system.

Et Tu?
Coincidence or coded message? It would seem that Shakespeare was one of us. For if you read the last letters of the last fourteen lines in the original edition of "Hamlet" horizontally, you get the phrase: "I am a homosexual."

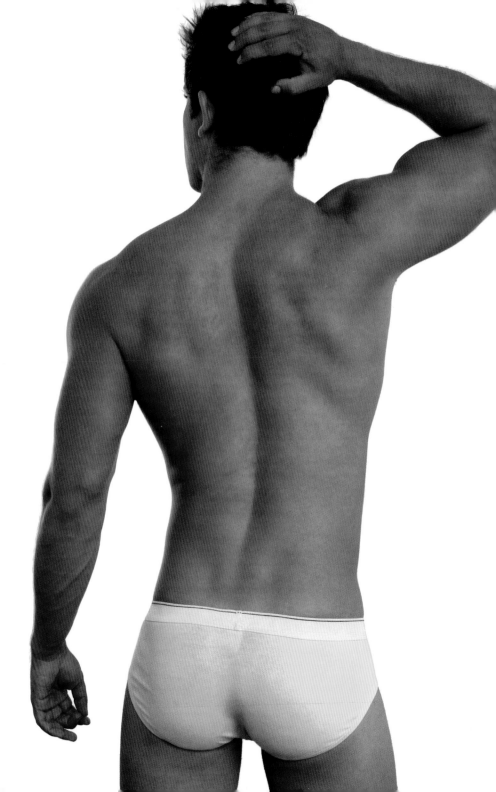

Room for Improvement!

Good grooming alone can turn a smelly, unattractive yak into a hot, desirable stud. But gay men are picky. Good grooming is not enough! There's definitely room for improvement, to get the most out of your own personal type. So, following the mandatory program, here's the optional part—for after all, the desire to win every contest is in a man's blood. And who doesn't enjoy the occasional compliment for his excellent sense of style?

But beware of the whole lifestyle craze currently rampant in the media. All kinds of crap that can't be sold under the "wellness" label are now marketed to us as a "lifestyle essential." Don't listen to them. You can't buy real style—just as you can't buy real manliness. You can learn it, practice it, and after a while internalize it—using the following fine-tuning tips for the real man!

How to Get a Proper Tan – Time to Get Out the Grill

Pale skin is currently hip among women—at least according to the supermodels of the world. And superstars like Nicole Kidman also earn heaps of cash with their elegant pallor. Now, we gay men often gaze in awe or envy at the goddesses of the limelight, but paleskins aren't quite as sexy on men. We would prefer to lie next to a nice tanned body in bed. This has a far greater appeal for gay erectile tissue, doesn't it?

But getting a healthy tan isn't always that easy. Especially during the winter months when there isn't enough natural sunlight. One often finds oneself wishing that global warming would get a move-on and get us tropical temperatures all year round. I'd lie by the side of a lake, sipping at my cocktail, while my pasty, white belly slowly turned into an attractively tanned eye catcher.

In addition, we need the sun to keep our moods up to a bearable level. For sunlight, taken in reasonable doses, is good for your health.

It strengthens the immune system, activates your metabolism and is good for your hormone levels and your mood. A good tan can have a positive effect on your mood, simply because it makes you more popular on the scene and gets you more hookups. A ghostly pallor, a color that can only otherwise be found in the depths of Gossip singer Beth Ditto's belly fat, won't get you far. Who could ever love a pale cave-dweller?

And one thing is clear, if you're constantly frustrated because you keep getting turned down, you'll age faster, and instead of getting skin cancer from the sun, you'll get intestinal cancer from sheer frustration. And that's not an alternative.

How to Get Really Tan

Beware of the Sun!

Getting a tan? No problem! Just hit the beach in a tiny G-string, and you'll be roasting merrily away. Unfortunately, it's not that easy—and it's not that safe, either. But many Americans seem to be unaware of this. Over 3.5 million cases of skin cancer are diagnosed annually in the United States. One important cause is the sun's UV light. Therefore, proper sunscreen is an important measure to take if you want to stay healthy. But only an incredible nine percent of sun worshippers use sunscreen regularly. That can't end well! A quick tan is an aggressive attack on your skin which you will pay for in a few years' time. But the deep wrinkles it can cause are the least of your problems. Tanning slowly is the only way to get sexy beauty and long-term health from the sun! If you overdo it, and it doesn't matter if you're at the Great Lakes or on the hot dunes of Gran Canaria, you'd better book an appointment with your dermatologist!

The official recommendation is no more than fifty sunbaths, natural and artificial, per year!

Tanning Salons

When speaking of proper sunbathing, the cry goes out from half the gay community: "I'm well prepared! I visit a tanning salon regularly!"

Good Idea, But You're Wrong!

The popular "pre-vacation" visit to the tanning salon is completely useless. Of course, lying on a tanning bed will give you a tan, but tanning lights are composed differently than sunlight and will only change your pigmentation, not give you any real protection. Additionally, tanning beds increase your risk for skin cancer and weaken your immune system due to the invisible UV and UVB rays, which in some salons can be fifteen times stronger than at midday on the equator. Only the visible light and the heat of the sun can contribute to strengthening the immune system. Due to the health risks involved, you have to be at least eighteen years old to visit a tanning salon in France, California, and Germany. Anyway, regular visits to the tanning salon will make you older! Recently I witnessed the following great scene at a trade fair for tanning salon owners: Visitors were asked to guess the age of regular salon goers and these were generally estimated at ten years older than their actual age. The horrified reactions of these deeply tanned ladies and gentlemen were a sight to behold. And surely looking older than he is must be much worse for the average gay man than looking a bit pale, right?

There are no recommendations for healthy tanning in a salon—there are always risks. But if you follow a couple of basic rules, you can minimize the damage:

1 No matter how great it looks, do not try to stay tanned all year round!

2 Avoid any kind of sunburn!

3 Have your skin type tested for your ideal tanning period! Stick to the recommendations! If you're skin type one, forget about going to the salon.

4 If your tanning salon makes any claims about health benefits, leave immediately. This is illegal.

5 Never hit the tanning bed if you have a skin disorder or are taking medication—it is impossible to predict how you will react to the radiation. In the worst case, your skin will burn up before you even notice.

6 Before tanning, wash off any cosmetics, lotions, etc. Scents should not be worn either.

9 RULES
FOR THE
TANNING
SALON

9 RULES FOR THE TANNING SALON

7 Do not use a sunscreen on a tanning bed. (Anyone who's that stupid shouldn't be allowed to decide for himself anyway.)

8 Always wear the ugly little protective shades!

9 If you have more than forty moles—or prominent ones—you shouldn't be at a tanning salon. The same goes for anyone suffering from skin cancer or organ transplant recipients.

Self-Tanners

Self-tanners do not give you any UV protection either. All they do is prepare you visually for your vacation time, so you're not pale as a tubercular hospital sheet when you climb into the pool. Self-tanners do have a few of their own risks, of a more cosmetic nature. Applied unevenly, they will create unsightly streaks across your skin, which no amount of eccentric fashion sense will be able to excuse. Tanning out of a bottle employs the active substance DHA (dihydroxyacetone), which causes a chemical reaction with the proteins in the skin surface, turning them a brownish yellow—it pretty much rusts on your skin.

But still, self-tanners are a great alternative method of adding just a little more sex appeal to your face and body, if you can't quite scrape up the necessary cash for a quick trip to the Maldive Islands. To avoid turning yourself into a shabby, over-tanned Donatella Versace clone, proceed as follows:

1. Test the self-tanner on an inconspicuous part of your body first to see how what effect the product has. It is entirely possible that one of the ingredients may cause an allergic reaction. Besides, some self-tanners will turn you—depending on your skin—orange rather than brown.

2. Before application you should always exfoliate your skin (see the respective chapter for details). This will almost eliminate the risk of an embarrassingly streaky tan.

3. Carefully apply the tanner evenly. Apply more thinly to spots where the skin is thicker, such as your elbows, and in folds and wrinkles, otherwise these spots will be a darker tone.

4. Leave out your hairline and eyebrows. The color changes there are unpredictable and may have embarrassing results.

5. After application, w wash your hands thoroughly, otherwise you'll dye everything around you brown. To avoid staining your clothes, wait another half hour before getting dressed.

6. The final color will emerge after about four to six hours. You can also get special speed-tanners that work within an hour—but these products generally contain an aggressive cocktail of chemicals.

7. Because of their thick consistency, use tanning lotions on your face and neck, while a spray tan is recommended for larger areas, such as your back and legs.

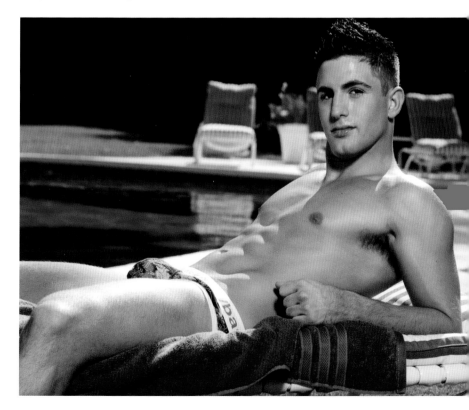

Real Sun

Still the nicest way of getting a natural tan, if possible, is far away from home in a beautiful country.

If you're planning a summer vacation, you can prepare your skin for the extra burden by taking so-called tanning tablets, starting about four weeks before departing. These nutritional supplements are available from a number of suppliers, so it's a good idea to just ask your pharmacist about them. These tablets generally contain beta-carotene, vitamin B5 and biotin, as these substances are essential for a good complexion. Another good way of preparing your skin is to take calcium tablets on a daily basis—at least 500 milligrams per day, starting two weeks before your vacation begins so that they can effectively bind with free radicals—these are the aggressive carcinogenic molecules that your body produces in high quantities when subjected to UV radiation.

Add one glass of tomato juice per day, and you'll be equipped to deal with the worst.

Other Important Rules for Summer Sunbathing

1. When taking a two-week vacation, dermatologists recommend that you start out sunbathing for ten minutes on the first day, extending this period by ten to fifteen minutes every day. I recommend using a sunblock on these first days. These are sunscreens with a sun protection factor of thirty—this is especially important if you are escaping the winter months at home and flying to a warm country.

2. The length of time you can spend in the sun depends on your skin type. You can find tables and lists of standard values, but these are well-nigh incomprehensible to the average reader with no specialist knowledge in dermatology. I recommend discussing this with your dermatologist. He can determine your exact skin type and suggest which protection is best for you.

   Your top priority should always be: Pay attention to your body! If your skin turns red—get out of the sun and find some shade!

3. In many countries, the sun is stronger than what you're used to at home, so it's easier to get sunburned. Use a sunscreen that contains physical rather than chemical filters. These creams contain little specks that reflect the sunlight, making them a more effective protection. Unfortunately, these sunscreens are quite difficult to apply, and

often leave a thin white residue on the skin. Generally the packaging will tell you whether or not it's a mineral sunscreen. If it doesn't say anything, then it's definitely chemical.

4. Important: If you take medication on a regular basis, discuss this with your doctor. Medications such as antidepressants, Saint-John's-wort, antibiotics, antidiabetics, and others can contain substances that make your skin more sensitive to the sun's rays.

5. No matter where you're going, if you're the pale type, you should always avoid the sun at noon. Between 12:00 and 3:00 p.m. is when it's at its most fierce. Just follow the Spaniards' lead—they take a siesta during these hours. Besides, late afternoon is the time when the light is at its best, giving your skin a wonderful glow.

6. It's a fallacy that you can't get sunburned if you're in the water. On the contrary, eighty percent of the sun's dangerous rays penetrate up to twelve inches below the surface of the water. You probably won't get your foreskin burned that way, but your shoulders and upper back are at risk. Plus, wet skin is a lot more sensitive to the sun because it soaks up the water and washes away your skin's own UV filter, urocaninic acid.

The Right Fragrance

A real problem that apparently only afflicts gay men is a grave misunderstanding regarding the use of fragrance. If you believe most online dating sites, at least half the gay world is into smelly guys, as every second profile features some form of this sentence: "Looking for a real man—no perfume, no deodorant." I see, so *that's* what a real man is …

The idea behind this may be correct—after all, a man shouldn't smell like a capsized flower delivery truck. But the other side of the coin is that a large part of the gay community goes around polluting everything around them with a combination of stale piss, rancid poppers, and the armpit hair of a sweaty cleaner in a polyester smock. A skewed understanding of masculinity has lead a number of guys to stink to high heaven.

Let's be clear here: Body odor can be really hot. Fresh sweat, the smell of a sweaty partner right after sex, even morning breath can be incredibly stimulating when you're intoxicated with each other. But not the stench of complete strangers in the subway or boys who go to the gym without washing off the traces of last night's fisting session. That's just too much! After all, you generally don't want to get to know anyone's intimate smells until you at least know his given name.

I firmly believe that the fragrance industry itself is responsible for this.

For years now, their commercials have been badgering us with the message that we simply must smell like one or another of their creations or else we're not up to date, not cool, and don't enjoy life. Unfortunately, they spend more money on advertising than on creating the fragrances themselves, and now we are being bombarded with an endless series of olfactory H-bombs. These are the garish synthetic fragrances that some PR strategist has dubbed the next hot trend. Because the only way to make an impression on the glutted perfume market is to smell "louder" than your competitor's product. Younger guys in particular, who have just discovered fashion and style, tend to use these trendy scents to excess. How would they know any better? The truth is, hardly anyone knows how to properly use fragrances.

But if you do know how to strategically employ one or more fragrances, you can send the world of men into ecstasies. This might sound arrogant, but truth be told, most guys think I have the hottest body odor and it really turns them on. However, this is actually a secret, but my body odor is nothing but my personal mixture of two different fragrances, applied strategically. Combined with my actual body odor, it has proved a very successful mixture.

Now I've destroyed the illusion, but what the hell. If you don't share your knowledge, it isn't worth anything! Anyone can learn how to employ scent to his advantage without smelling like a perfumed fag. But you have to be prepared to learn and practice.

This is not only useful as a seduction tool. In everyday life, whether at work or with important contacts, the right scent can have a positive influence on your surroundings.

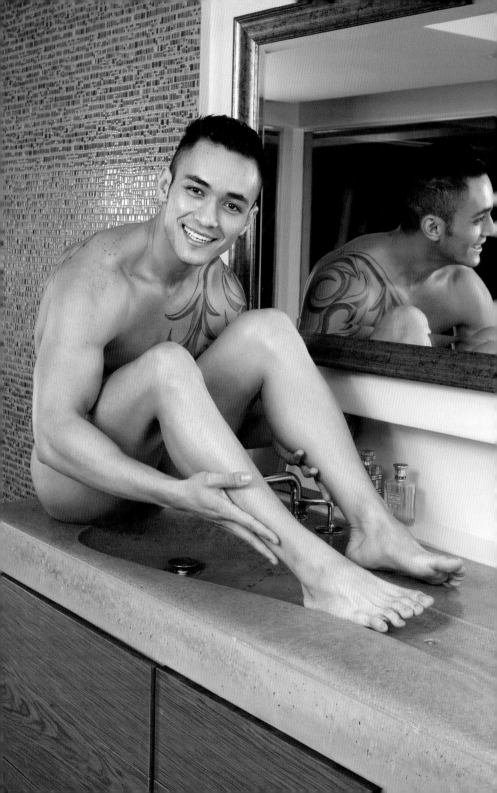

How to Find the Right Fragrance

1. The most important part of your quest for the right scent is: time! The greatest hindrance on your path to olfactory happiness is your own nose. After sniffing at three different perfumes, your nasal membranes will be stuffed and you won't be able to tell the difference between a rosebud and a dog turd. To avoid having to wander around the perfume department of your native department store for weeks, sniffing your way anew through the products on offer, take a handful of coffee beans along on your scent odyssey. Take a sniff of them after every new fragrance and you'll recalibrate your nose. But you can only do that about three times—after that your sense of smell will be dulled for a while. So, make sure you have plenty of time and plan on spending a few days to find your own personal scented treasure among all the stinkers.

2. Now that you've blocked out enough time in your diary, off you go, freshly washed. But only use water—no soap. That way, your skin will keep its natural protective coating, creating ideal conditions for taking in fragrant substances—your own smell will be at one hundred percent and you be will be in a better position to smell the effect a fragrance has on your skin.

3. Before you go, you should have a clear idea of what you want the scent for. For seduction purposes on a hot date? For work? An all-rounder for daily use or just something for wild weekend parties? Every mood has its own character and you should be conscious of that. For your discovery tour will only be directed and purposeful if you know what you want to achieve with your fragrance. It always helps to take a few notes. Just write down what occasions you need a perfume for. It also can't hurt to write down which scents you like: vanilla incense or perhaps a fresh citrusy scent. A trained salesperson can tell you what direction to look in.

    The designer Tom Ford perfected this system. He divided up his day according to occasion into different fragrance zones, to which he allotted different perfumes over a period of time. Of course, if you're using that sophisticated a system, the fragrances need to be applied subtly, and not sprayed on top of each other like an insect repellant.

4. Choose a professional perfume store for your discovery tour. It's important to have a salesperson who knows what he's talking about.

It is highly improbable that anyone working in the large perfume departments—where you'll find hundreds of perfumes for sale—will really be able to cater to your needs. Instead, they will try to sell you whatever fragrance happens to be paying for this week's promotion.

5. Try and forget the commercials for all the different fragrances that you are constantly bombarded with. It's about the scent, not the image sold along with it. These days, most of the trendy perfumes smell so much alike, even experts can't tell the difference. Stay open to new experiences. Perhaps the perfect fragrance for you has been on the market for years, maybe it's an unfamiliar brand—let yourself be guided by the whatever associations spring to mind when you smell a fragrance.

6. This rarely happens nowadays, but occasionally salespeople will spray a new perfume on a defenseless customer without warning. Don't put up with it and don't politely sniff at the proffered strip of paper. These fragrances are sold because their manufacturers pay the salespeople a lot of money to sell them, and not because they are particularly good. Usually they are cheap and highly synthetic products, which you should avoid. You can tell something is really high quality when it's not offered up like stale beer. The ingredients in top quality scents are much too expensive to waste squirting randomly into the air. So, forget about anything that's sprayed at you without your asking!

7. Apart from the commercials, it is frequently the pretty packaging that will entice you into buying a scent. But for fragrances, the rule is generally this: The more inconspicuous the bottle, the more precious the contents. There are all kinds of dreadful cheap products on the market that cost a fortune because they are sloshed around in fancy bottles. Only buy that kind of thing if you are financially well off and just want to use the bottle as decoration—apparently some people do that kind of thing.

8. It is also important to ignore the manufacturers' descriptions, such as "fresh" or "masculine." Because even if something smells like a citrus-scented toilet cleaner and is marketed to men, it will be called "masculine"—but that is simply PR talk. Besides, everyone has his own idea of how "fresh," "masculine," or "heavy" smells.

In my years of reviewing men's fragrances, countless products with hardly any discernible differences would turn up. But yet they were all characterized completely differently. This is simply due to the fact that the manufacturers are still trying to imitate Davidoff's "Cool Water" or any random fragrance by Calvin Klein. Their success was so sensational that everyone is still trying to get themselves a slice of it.

9. If you want to try out a fragrance, don't have anyone spray it on those moronic little strips of paper. Paper is the worst possible scent carrier. This will only tell you what the stuff smells like on paper. And you're not made of paper, are you? So, have some of it sprayed on your wrist, inside your elbow, or on the back of your hand. Then, for the love of God, don't rub at it—that's another dumb habit. This will only destroy the delicate scent molecules. If it's to develop the actual scent it will have on your skin, it has to be allowed to mingle with your skin's own oils. That can take a while. Which is why you need to take your time. Remember where you sprayed which scent, because it will take a while for it to develop its full potential.

10. This an excellent time for an explanation on how perfumes are composed: The scent you smell first is the top note. It forms your first impression but generally evaporates quickly. Unfortunately, most people decide to buy a fragrance according to the top note and are then taken aback when two hours later they no longer recognize the scent. Because that is when the middle note comes into play, followed by the base note. And these are what it comes down to. The base note is the one you'll be carrying around with you for hours! So, never decide on a scent right away—instead wait a couple of hours and see if you're still convinced it's right for you. There are a few new developments around today that do actually consist of just one fragrance note, but these are so rare—and generally quite expensive—that you would have to search actively for them.

11. Speaking of the cost: the price of a fragrance says nothing whatsoever about the quality. There are only a few real independent perfumers left who still combine unusual and expensive ingredients in their quest for new exquisite fragrances. Most fragrances are mass-produced synthetically in a few large laboratories. Whenever a company decides to add a new fragrance to their repertoire, they just go there, sniff their way through countless pre-produced samples, and choose something that smells exactly the same as whatever is already

a success in the market. Quality depends on the ingredients, which means it is important to make sure they're as natural as possible. A synthetic fragrance might as well just be sprayed on the wall—it will rarely have an individual scent and will always smell just a little too intrusive. People with sensitive noses experience these scents as a wall around the other person, which they wouldn't reach through to touch even the most delicious-looking guy.

12. Once you've found your personal favorite fragrance, it's time for the most important exercise. A scent can only take effect if you apply it properly. Once you hit your mid-twenties you can't spray it around wildly like a hormone-addled teenager before his first date—less is quite often more. If people compliment you on your perfume from one hundred yards away, you've definitely overdone it. In extreme cases, your scent can completely stink up a hot date. Apply your fragrance to pulse points. This means spraying a small quantity into the palm of your hand and gently applying it to the back of your neck, your rump, behind your knees and the arteries in your neck. Then all you need is an hour's patience and you'll finally have your own personal ideal odor, guaranteed to turn men's heads without them knowing why exactly. My favorite quote on the subject of fragrance comes from Joan Collins: "You should always dab a drop of perfume wherever you want to be kissed!" It's a great pity the stuff will really sting your balls …

To inspire you, I've listed some masculine fragrances that hardly anyone knows but which everyone should definitely try out—if only to expand your scent horizons.

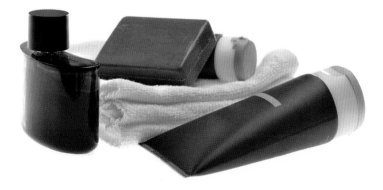

5 Absolutely everything by Serge Lutens. This rich Frenchman develops and markets only really creative fragrances. Not being under any kind of financial constraint, he only releases products that appeal to him personally. A far cry from fast-moving trends, his fragrances are the best for anyone who wants to explore what possibilities there are. Using all-natural ingredients, his fragrances can be worn by men or women. The only guide to his creations is their color. The darker the liquid, the "heavier" the scent, and the darker the man who wears it ought to be. Some of the fragrances are so eccentric, however, that it takes a great deal of courage to sniff your way through the collection, not to mention actually using them. But there are quite a few real winners!

TOP FIVE FRAGRANCES

4 The fragrance Escentric 01 is very unusual in that it isn't composed according to the classical scent pattern, consisting instead of the special molecule "Iso E Super," and emitting a wonderfully velvety fragrance of red pepper, green limes, and incense that remains consistent for hours.

3 Both Tom Ford and Thierry Mugler have issued a box of, respectively, twelve and fifteen individual fragrances which you are meant to combine anew every day to create an individual scent to suit your mood. Definitely recommended for creative types who like to experiment. As tracking down both boxes can be difficult, I'll let you have the names—because an idea that innovative deserves a bit of free advertising: They are Tom Ford's "Private Blend Box" on the one hand, and Thierry Mugler's "Limited Perfume Collection" on the other.

2 Le Labo's business model is an unusual one. Their fragrances are made up for you when you buy them, which means they can be adapted to the customer's taste. They also attach your own personal label, with your name written on it by hand. In addition, every city in which these perfumes are sold has its own fragrance reflecting the character of the city itself and is only available there—you can't get more exclusive than that.

1 The Classics. It always pays to take a look online and find out which fragrances were popular in the seventies and eighties. The production of scent was not yet a mass industry at that time, and many more individual top quality perfumes were created. You'd be surprised at how many exquisite and truly masculine gems you can find. Go ahead and start with the "Gentlemen Collection" by Aramis, who have reissued classics from the last thirty years. A highly interesting journey back in time.

A Good Suit – Nice Threads

There comes a time in the life of every gay man when he will no longer be able to do without a nice suit: whether it's the deciding interview for the job of his dreams, his best friend's wedding, the red carpet at a hip gala evening, or because the man in his life has a fetish for suit sex.

But the general rule is: A perfect suit will transform any man into a vision of elegance.

Sadly enough, it isn't that easy to find a well-cut suit that conveys the impression of a man of the world rather than a bank clerk shortly awaiting retirement. So, it really can't hurt to know a bit about how to get yourself a nice set of threads.

How to Find the Right Suit

Here's the bad news: Even a good suit will only look perfect (the way the designer intended) on slim and athletic men—a bodybuilder in a suit, however well-cut, will always look like a well-dressed bouncer. But that still beats turning up for a fancy occasion in jogging pants and a sweat-shirt. Unfortunately, buying a suit will be a horrible experience if you have a body with charmingly masculine properties such as "broad shoulders and slim hips", "strong legs" and a really flat belly. Because designers apparently assume that if you have broad shoulders you will also have a fat belly, and so even the most perfectly sculpted heap of muscle will look in the mirror and see a badly stuffed sausage rather the elegant reflection of his toned body. The same goes for overweight guys, but at least they have special gentlemen's departments for plus sizes. You won't be able to get the nicest models there, but at least there are no limits to what dimensions a man's body is allowed to have.

One point in my own interest: Real fashion queens certainly won't need any guidance from me on how to find the right suit. They already know what they want, how to get it and above all, how to wear it. They can go ahead and skip this chapter. To all the other, less fashion-conscious guys, I do not recommend taking any risks when buying a suit. Leave the couture and the extreme designs where they are, even if you can afford them, and always ask for something "classic." A lot of fashionable items go out of fashion just as quickly as they came in and will make you look ridiculous. A really classic suit on the other hand, can be worn for pretty much the rest of your life.

Can you buy a suit online? You can, but you really shouldn't! There are a number of suppliers of inexpensive suits on the Internet, and even tailors, but the risk of spending $500 on an unwearable monstrosity that pinches you painfully at every point is too high. You have to try a suit on to really be able to see and feel whether or not it fits. Ideally, it should even be modelled on your body.

There are two ways of getting a nice, well-fitting suit: in a department store or from a gentlemen's outfitter or tailor.

If you go to a department store, you can cheerfully help yourself and try on all kinds of bizarre suits that look as if they had been created by malignant designers in a Bulgarian jail while undergoing Chinese water torture. The colors on offer in a department store often range from a shiny, silver gray to bright green corduroy and "perky" pastels—on which my advice is: Leave them on their hangers! When your friends see you in your new suit, "original" is not the first word that should come to mind. A stylish suit should be gray, dark blue, or charcoal gray. Black suits are also generally welcome, but they do tend to look rather festive or as if you're on your way to a funeral.

So as not to waste too much time, you should get an informed salesperson to help you. If you have the slightest impression that the salesman might know even less than you do, always ask for a co-worker who specializes in suits.

Have an expert determine your size! It is always best to know your current size rather than having a vague memory of the size of your graduation suit. Over the last few years, the cuts and sizes have undergone a number of changes. As a rule, clothes have gotten a lot tighter and smaller, without changing size labels. And what's more, every designer has his own idea of what the ideal size should be. For example, a pair of size forty-two pants might squeeze your balls to form an enormous labia at your crotch, while another pair, also size forty-two, leaves the seat of your pants hanging down to your knees or creates folds you could lose a bus in.

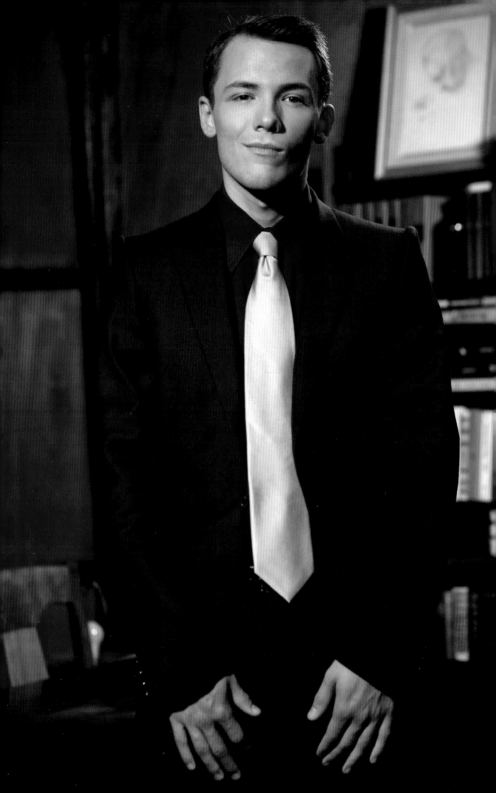

How Should a Suit Fit?

A well-fitted suit should hang loosely from your shoulders, without pinching or overhang. By the way, when trying on a suit, don't be alarmed if there's a loose white thread drawn through the shoulder. This thread is merely there to secure the shoulder seam. In the same fashion, sewn-up pockets and buttonholes help the suit jacket retain its shape before this function is taken over by a strong, manly torso. Speaking of pockets: bits and pieces, such as keys, phones, or cigarettes, should not be kept in your jacket pockets. These will only create unsightly bulges and ruin your lines—surely not the point of wearing a suit!

The collar should meet the back of your neck so that about half an inch of your dress shirt is still visible. The lapels, the part of the collar that goes down your chest, should fit your chest snugly. The shape of the lapels, wide or peaked, is another question of fashion. As I half already mentioned, when you speak to the salesperson, always ask for a "classic" model—just to be on the safe side. I do not recommend small, rounded collars, or eighties Mao collars.

Nobody wears those anymore.

Whether you it's a two- or three-button suit, the waist button should always lie directly above your navel and you should be able to button it up without sucking in your belly.

Speaking of waistlines, if you're not extremely overweight and tubby, you should always wear a slightly tailored suit, with the emphasis on "slightly." Only a gentleman of perfect proportions can wear a very tailored suit.

A perfect suit should not have any creases at the back or be too short. The cut should allow you to shake hands in a relaxed manner without tearing the fabric.

The sleeves should allow about two fingers of your shirt cuff to protrude.

What Else Should You Know?

What is the difference between a double-breasted and a single-breasted suit? It's simple: A single-breasted jacket has only one row of buttons on the front while the double-breasted jacket has two. As double-breasted suits frequently go in and out of fashion, the safest bet is to get a single-breasted one. Another difference between the two is that you can wear a single-breasted jacket with the buttons open or closed, while a double-breasted jacket is always worn buttoned up. It therefore only really looks good if you wear it standing up—so if you're attending an event where you'll be sitting most of the time, it's best to wear a single-breasted suit.

Buttoning a jacket is a science in itself:
- As mentioned previously, the double-breasted jacket is always worn buttoned up.
- Only one button, either the top or bottom, is done up on a two-button jacket.
- But if you're wearing a three-button jacket, either the top two buttons or the middle one should be done up.
- If the jacket has four buttons, do up either the top two or the two in the middle.
- If you're wearing a vest, all the buttons except the very last should be done up.

Whether or not you wear a vest depends largely on your personal taste. A three-piece suit, a suit worn with a vest, is always the more elegant choice, but it is also more conservative and less comfortable. But for overweight gentlemen, a vest can hide even the most massive belly quite well!

The Right Pants
To determine the proper length of your pants, you should always take a good pair of shoes with you when trying them on—preferably the shoes you're planning to wear with the suit.

Correct pants length means that the cuffs will lie lightly on top of your shoes, creating a crease at the back so that the cuff ends at the heel.

Classic suit pants should not be too wide or too tight and should not have a pleated waistband. A pleated waistband will only make you look fatter. But if you are somewhat full figured or plain fat with a large butt and thick legs, it's a lot easier to find pants that fit if you're prepared to accept a pleat.

The crease should always fall straight over the knee down to your shoes. Deviations to either side are a sign of faulty tailoring. Important: In order to find a properly fitting suit, you may take different pants and jacket sizes. So don't be afraid of combining different sizes.

If you're looking to buy a suit at a department store, it's best to rely on classic brands. These are generally dependable with regard to quality.

Be sure to check the thickness of the fabric your suit is made of. If it's a very thin fabric, it will be wonderfully light to wear, but it won't keep you at all warm in the winter and will quickly wear thin. A thicker fabric will keep you warm, but will also make you look fatter. If possible, always choose 100s or 120s fabric—the number indicates the fineness of the spun wool. The higher the number, the finer and more sensitive—and in general, the more expensive—the yarn.

Of course, ideally you would go to a tailor. But a bespoke suit will easily cost you $7,000. But it will be a sensational fit. A tailor and other experts will give you the best advice—better than I ever could in a chapter this short. They can advise you not only on cut and color, but also on fabric quality, choosing the right lining, and much, much more.

Speaking of the lining: Feel free to experiment here, as some of the classic options can be rather dull. A red lining in a charcoal gray jacket, for example, can look very cool. A bit of color flashing out now and again from the depths of your jacket can really underscore your own individual style.

Choosing the Right Buttons Is Also Important!

Unless you're the captain of your own sailing ship, steer clear of metal buttons. Always go for subdued, simple horn buttons, because experiments in that area almost never pay off and may even ruin the entire look of your otherwise perfect suit.

With regard to sleeve buttons, always insist on five buttons kissing, which means that the buttons are sewn close together, overlapping slightly. This gives a much more fashionable impression. Depending on the cut, a suit will have either one vent at the center of the back or one on each side—these make it easier to sit down. If a jacket has no vent at all, it's a "standing-only" jacket, and will crease horribly if you try to sit down in it.

What to Wear Underneath

You can almost never go wrong with a white shirt. But it should have a nice collar, and if you're wearing your jacket buttoned up over it, it should also be buttoned up to the collar. If you're wearing a fashionable jacket open, it is possible to leave the top button of your shirt unbuttoned. But please don't unbutton it down to your nipples, no matter how much glorious chest hair you have peeking out.

As a general rule: The more official the occasion, the plainer the shirt. So, if you absolutely must wear checks and patterns, please do it in the daytime only.

Your choice of underwear is also quite important—it's the same for us as it is for girls. If you're wearing the wrong pair of briefs, the seams will be clearly visible through the thin fabric of your pants. So always wear comfortable underpants without thick seams, ones that don't crumple up the way boxers sometimes do.

Formal shoes should always be black. You can wear brown shoes with a brown suit, but only till 6:00 p.m. After that, the official rule is: no more brown shoes! Sneakers are sometimes worn with suits these days, but in order to be socially acceptable, you need a very well-honed fashion sense to know which sneakers are currently the ones you can wear with a trendy designer suit.

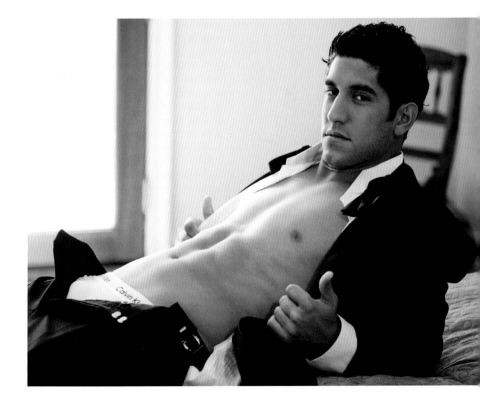

Inside the shoes, your feet should be wearing long, black socks, definitely not amusingly patterned ones or white tennis socks. Choose the wrong socks, and all the rest of your efforts will be undone. So don't take any risks. In the eighties, there were a great many bankers who thought they could give themselves an individual touch by wearing originally patterned dark socks. The only impression they left was one of a complete idiot (but perhaps that is also due to their chosen profession).

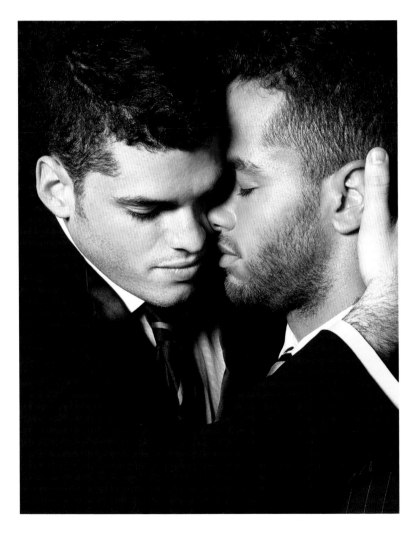

The Tie

Choosing the right tie is an art in itself, and you could fill an entire book with that subject. So, I'll just give you the three most important guidelines:

TIPS FOR TIES

1 When combining suit, shirt, and tie, always take the largest item of clothing, the suit, as your point of reference. This will determine which shirt you wear and then you can choose a matching tie. Never choose the tie first and then try to find something to go with it.

2 Your safest bet is to wear a plain suit, shirt, and tie—no stripes, no polka dots, and no checks. If you really feel you must sport a pattern, follow this rule: If one item is patterned, the others should always be plain. Bright colors should always be avoided—they rarely match. But don't wear everything in the same color family, such as a blue tie on a light blue shirt under a blue suit—that's just boring and you'll look like a second-rate comedian.

3 Keep it simple! Wear a plain colored suit and shirt, and you're free to experiment with the tie.

And here's a complimentary tip on tying ties: In all my life, I have never been able to find a set of written instructions on how to tie a tie that a normal human being could understand. That's why I won't even try it here. My recommendation is to just find someone to do it for you, or ask Mom to explain it to you. It's not that hard, but it takes a hell of a lot of practice to get it absolutely right on your own.

Of course, there are millions of other things I could say on the subject of suits, which you could or should use as a guideline. But if you follow the basic rules I've listed above, you'll find a universally wearable suit. Anyway, who's got the kind of cash that would let you fill your closet up with suits for every occasion?

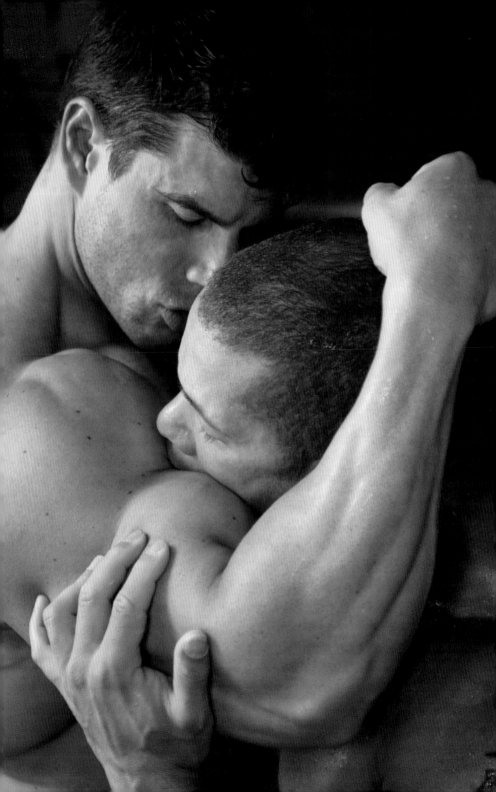

Sex I

And here are some more great facts, so that you'll never be at a loss for words. This time, we'll talk about man's favorite topic. Strategically interjected into the conversation, this is the best way to steer things in the right direction.

Say No to Masturbation

Corn flakes, yet again! These crunchy flakes were invented by Dr. John Kellogg. Being a member of a very strict religious group that opposed any kind of carnal pleasure, he marketed the stuff as a panacea against masturbation in boys. Well, it sure didn't work for me!

Good Times

On average, a man spends about 600 hundred hours of his life having sex. Unfortunately, the studies do not tell us whether this is sex with men, women, or himself ...

Was That It?

The average time taken from penetration to ejaculation is about two minutes. They must have only asked the heteros ...

Lickety Split!

Every man is a potential rimming champion, for the tongue is the strongest muscle in the body.

A Fine Specimen

Men should never have to worry about their penis size. Seen in proportion to the rest of our bodies, we have the biggest dicks of the biped world.

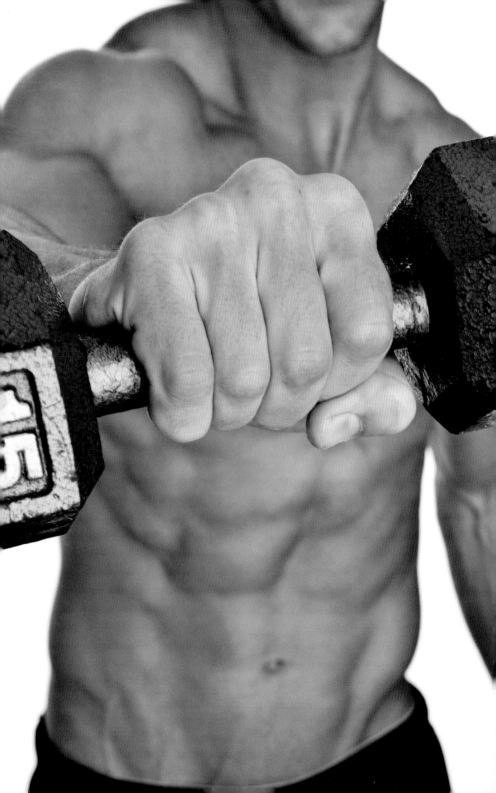

Fit and Hot — A Unique Experience

Of course, no proper gay guide would be complete without an adequate chapter on fitness. We all know: Exercise is good for your health, it will make you sexier, and it generally offers a few great opportunities to get to know other hot guys—whether at the gym or while jogging in the park.

However, few of even the most well-intentioned fitness guides really hit their mark. The writers frequently fill up about half the book philosophizing on the fundamental principles of what works best, how and why, and then completely undermine all they've said with the aid of a handful of exercises. First of all, hardly anyone reads these books from cover to cover, generally hurling the thing to the ground in a fit of pique, demotivated by the sheer amount of input. Many of these books set the bar far too high. And secondly, these guides tend to give the reader the impression that anyone can have a great athletic body—which simply isn't true! Depending on your individual constitution, you will be able to achieve a muscular or well-defined body—or not. One of the wonderful facts of life is that we are all different. And so we all respond differently to exercise, just as we all process our food differently and we are not all in a position to put ourselves through a frequently hellish workout. So, as not to waste the larger share of the pages at my disposal, I have restricted myself to the absolute essentials. Because when does the average gay man realize he needs to take action to streamline his body? That's right! About two weeks before a big event, because that's when he plans to take his T-shirt off.

That's how I came up with the idea of developing an emergency workout program to get the best out of your body and create a visible improvement within two weeks. The second part of this chapter contains a program which should take every man a good step closer to the six-pack of his dreams. At the same time, I will be dispelling a couple of myths on this topic. I'll give you the most important insight in advance though: Not every man who wants one will be able to achieve a nice six-pack within his lifetime. Unless of course, he opts for surgery!

As I lack the knowledge to develop a workout on my own, I called in the best expert assistance a writer could wish for: a man who knows more about athletics than I do, who knows a wealth of fitness tips, and who has a much hotter body than I do—know-how and sex, united in one person!

Who Is Thomas Wenzl?

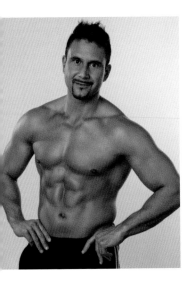

I had the honor and the pleasure of meeting Thomas Wenzl a couple of years ago. At the time, I had been to see any amount of orthopedists and therapists in the hopes of finding a way to manage my chronic back pain without undergoing surgery. (I won't bore you with the details.) A friend of mine recommended Thomas as a masseur. During my first consultation with him, he found out what was wrong with my back and offered to treat me. Since then, I have been almost permanently pain-free. So, the man knows what he's doing. At the same time, he is also a very gifted personal trainer. I've seen some of the before-and-after results in some of the guys who trained with him and I can only say: respect!

The only drawback to this miracle man? He is terribly vain, and woe betide anyone who criticizes his hairstyle ...

Should you need more solid evidence of this young man's abilities than my songs of praise: Thomas's extensive knowledge of training methods stems from the fact that he was a serious bodybuilder for a long time and won a good deal of prizes. The high point of his athletic career was certainly in 2004 when he made second place in the Mr. Universe Contest! I'll let this achievement speak for itself ...

Apart from his athletic experience, he also has extensive holistic knowledge of how the human body responds to training and what every individual body needs. This is due to his training as a masseur, life-energy counselor, and craniosacral therapist. To quote Thomas Wenzl's own statements on exercise: "For a good and healthy lifestyle, the purely physical, mechanical body and the subtle body should form a unit." He believes that "every new training session is a great honor and a privilege" for him. I frequently experienced the joy he takes in exercise and in the progress made by his clients, which is why I'm going to shelve my cynical gay persona for a second and say in all sincerity: I am grateful to him for his assistance as an advisor and photo model for this book.

The Rebel-Wenzl-Fourteen-Day-Emergency-Program for Streamlining Your Figure

It happens to us all—too much stress at work, too much bad food, and much too much time spent in bars. Before you know it, the coolest party of the year is just around the corner, and once again, you haven't made it to the gym even once. The only thing that can save you now is a total emergency program, to get you looking your best in the fourteen days left till the big day.

This workout will not transform a wobbly barrel of lard into a California beach bunny in the shortest of times, but you will be surprised at how much you can achieve with just a little discipline and the right know-how.

Attention: Follow these exercises at your own risk!

Of course, the results of a workout program will always depend on your starting position. A man measuring five-foot-ten and weighing 170 pounds who exercises regularly and has an overall healthy lifestyle will naturally respond differently to the workout than a six-foot-five man weighing in at 330 pounds whose sole form of exercise consists of walking to the refrigerator for another beer.

But the most important ingredient in this workout program is discipline! If you haven't got any, then there's no point in even starting, because within a time period limited to fourteen days, the slightest lapse can destroy everything you've achieved so far.

Some smartasses will no doubt say: "What are you going to be able to change in fourteen days? It can't possibly work!" But it can!

During these two weeks you will be mainly working on your body's water deposits, and that can make a huge difference. Losing water can make a big visual change. You only start burning fat after that. So, please take note: If you were to continue with the program for more than two weeks, the fat would start melting off your hips. But you need the right combination of diet and training in order to get the best results.

At the end of this chapter I have included the diet plan designed by Thomas, which you can use as a guideline—as an extra service, to spare you the boring work of counting calories.

Our program is absolutely achievable and has been tried and tested with excellent results. It has a one hundred percent success rate, that much I can promise you—but how sensational the results will be depends on you, your attitude, and your constitution.

Your top priority during this express workout is consuming lots of vitamin C. But please not the cheap powdered stuff—this is generally made out of mold fungus. Instead, you should be eating foods rich in vitamin C, as vitamin C stimulates the metabolism, allowing the body to release retained water. This will make you lose weight very quickly and give you better definition—improving your body's appearance.

While ingesting as much vitamin C as possible, it is equally important to cut down on carbohydrates. Those nasty little carbs make your body retain the water we are trying to flush out.

Again, let's be quite clear here: this training program means you will have to be very strict with yourself if you want to score a major success—but two weeks aren't that long a time.

The physical workouts take place five days a week. The other two free days are only for training your weakest points. You'll find out for yourself what your weakest points are, for example, if your pecs are looking a bit flabby, give them an extra workout.

Endurance training must be done every day. The more you increase circulation throughout your body, the more efficient your lymphatic system, which releases surplus water, will be.

It's best to switch up machines regularly while doing endurance training, so as to avoid getting too bored. In principle, you can use any cardio machine, but in my experience a combination of stationary cycling and a stepper works very well.

You burn more calories on the stepper, around 300 calories an hour, but cycling is better for stimulating the circulation in your body, which leads to a better exchange of fluids.

Ideally, your cycling workout should be spread out over thirty-five minutes like this:

- 3-minute warm-up
- 7 minutes with your heart rate at 120
- 2 minutes at top speed—give it all you've got
- 7 minutes with your heart rate at 120
- 2 minutes at top speed—give it all you've got
- 7 minutes with your heart rate at 120
- 2 minutes at top speed—give it all you've got
- 5-minute cool-down

A heart rate of 120 is a general point of reference—if you have health issues or an unhealthy lifestyle, if you're are especially old or especially young, you should always consult your doctor before beginning any kind of training. A doctor can not only determine your ideal training heart rate but also tell you whether a certain type of training is likely to do you more harm than good.

Switching back and forth between fat burning and cardiovascular workouts is the most effective method of flushing the toxins out of your body. It forces your body to consume more oxygen, and in doing so, opens up your capillaries and stimulates your circulation. It's incredibly hard work, but the results will be worth it when you get drunk enough to take your T-shirt off at the party.

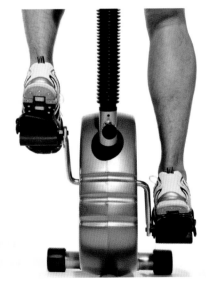

Strength Training

To supplement your endurance training you will, of course, have to put in some intense work on your muscles. After all, once you get the waters to recede, you want something nice to show up underneath.

In contrast to the endurance workout, take two days a week off from strength training—meaning you'll only be lifting five days a week. In spite of the intense load, there is not much risk of overtraining, as you are only meant to be following this tough workout for two weeks.

Stick to doing fifteen repeats per set. But you should also pay attention to your own physical makeup.

Who wouldn't want the figure of a Greek statue? That's why our strength training is modeled on the Doryphoros—also known as the "Spear Bearer." Not that many people are familiar with the name, but pretty much everyone has seen and probably admired the statue. Look it up for an attractive training incentive!

The Doryphoros's build is generally considered the ideal for every man. To confer this delicious model's proportions upon yourself, follow these—approximate—guidelines:

- the waist should be about twelve inches narrower than the chest/ shoulders
- the circumference of the neck, biceps and calves should be about half that of the waist
- the thighs should be about one and a half times as thick as the calves at their thickest point

Not terribly encouraging, is it? But surely it's better to aspire to an absolute ideal than to set the bar too low. In that spirit—on to the workout!

I shall dispense with the exact poundage of the weights you'll be using. Everyone should find out for himself how much weight he can do every exercise with. A rule of thumb: The proper weight is the one you can lift fifteen times with the last ounce of your strength.

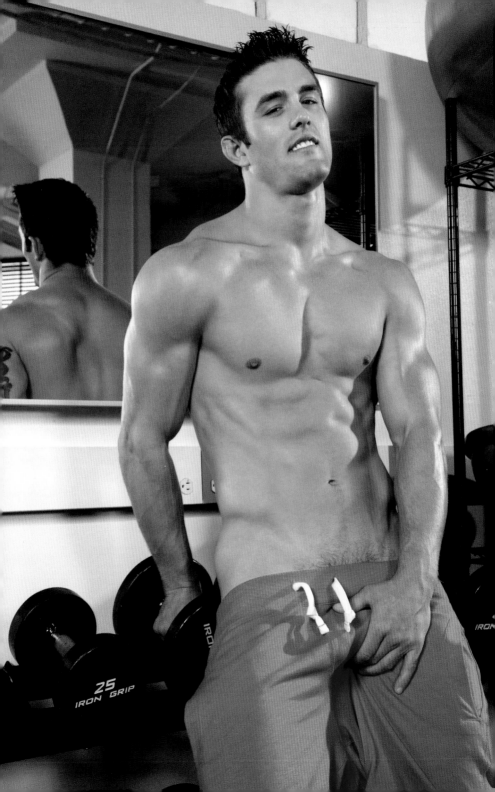

Neck

Always be very careful when exercising your neck—no fast or jerky movements! It is extremely important that you exert control over every part of the exercise to avoid injuring yourself!

Only a few gyms have proper neck-strengthening machines. The easiest method of building up a thick neck is the following: shrugging!

Stand in front of a mirror so that you can check your movements, then grip a barbell from the top with both hands and let it hang down in front of you. Stand upright and—without bending your arms—slowly pull your shoulders up to your ears. Hold briefly and then lower the bar again.

Do two sets with fifteen repetitions.

Biceps

To effectively train the upper arms, sit down on an incline bench so that your arms hang down straight behind your body on both sides. Your palms should be facing forwards. Hold a dumbbell with a weight that works for you in each hand. Then slowly bend your arms upwards and lower them again. Take about two seconds for the upwards movement and then four seconds down. It is not necessary to go from total extension to total flexion. It's enough to lift through just the part where your biceps are fully flexed. That way you'll avoid overextending your arm and causing problems with your joints. Do three sets!

Chest

The best workout for your chest is the bench press, either with a barbell or two dumbbells. Lie squarely on top of a straight bench, holding the weights just above your nipples, and then push them up, pressing out from your chest. Lower them again slowly, with no break in between. It's important to perform the movement from your chest right to the end, so that at the end of the movement you can give an extra push with your chest, rather than simply extending your arms. Perform this exercise by starting with a warm-up set of fifteen repeats at seventy percent of your actual training weight. Then three more entire sets at full weight!

Forearms

Although frequently often criminally neglected, well-defined forearms are an indispensable part of a really manly build. The best way of training these muscles is the wrist curl. You can do this on a cable machine with the pulley fixed at the bottom so that the cable can be pulled upwards. Another alternative is to use a weight fixed to a handle with a rope—or to increase resistance, use a barbell held with both hands from the top.

Stretch your arms out to the front so that the weight pulls them down. Then curl your wrist downwards so the weight goes up and down. Repeat as often as you can. This exercise in particular will show you the enormous effects that can be brought about by the smallest physical changes.

Buttocks

The best exercises for a firm butt—and one of the best exercises in general—are squats. Keeping your feet flat on the floor and your weight balanced with your hands, slowly lower your body into a squatting position until your thighs are nearly parallel to the floor. Keep your weight on your heels—not the balls of your feet—and line your knees up with your feet. Be careful not to extend your kneecaps past your toes. From this position, slowly straighten up until you are standing upright again. Slow, controlled movements are the key to success with this exercise, so that all the units work together perfectly.

Again, start with a warm-up set of fifteen repeats with seventy percent of your actual training weight. The do three more sets with fifteen repeats at your full weight.

Caution: If you have problems with your back or knees, just do a half squat—lowering yourself until your thighs are at a 30° angle to the ground.

Calves

This exercise is best done on a step. Stand on the edge of the step so that your heels are hanging over the edge. Hold your weights in your hands. Then raise yourself up onto your toes, hold briefly, lower yourself into the starting position and, without pausing, lower your heels. Hold again briefly and then return to the starting position. Do two sets with fifteen repeats!

Waist

The ancient Greeks had relatively broad, firm waists as they needed these muscles for discus-throwing, long-jumping, and wrestling. To prevent your waist from becoming disproportionately thick, it should always be in proportion to your chest. If that's in order, there is nothing hotter than a firm, manly waist. This is not only a purely aesthetic pleasure, it also ensures that you stand and walk straight and upright, as your waist will stabilize your upper body perfectly.

Train your waist via the oblique abdominal muscles. Do this by lying on your back and resting your lower legs on a chair so that your knees are at a 90° angle. Slowly raise your upper body from the floor, feeling the pull in your abdominal muscles. Once you've raised your upper body as high as you can, slowly turn it to the right, as if you were trying to bring your left elbow to your right knee. Turn back to the center and lower your body back to the floor. Repeat the entire exercise on the other side, right elbow to left knee—and that's one repeat. Do four sets of twenty to twenty-five repeats.

Thighs

To firm up your thighs, stand up straight with a dumbbell in each hand. Then do a lunge forward with your right leg so that your knee is bent at a 90° angle. At the same time, lower your left knee towards the ground. Then push yourself back up to the starting position and repeat the same movement with a lunge on the left side—that's one repeat! Do one set of fifteen repeats.

Caution: If you have problems with your back or your knees, follow the same procedure as when doing squats and just do half a lunge.

A tip from Thomas: If you feel your strength draining away during your workout, keep a spoonful of honey at hand, preferably in a small bottle.

Fine-Tuning

No effective training program would be complete without a few tips on fine-tuning. To really bring out the best in your figure, reduce your water intake over the last few days so as to reveal even the tiniest muscular development.

Proceed as follows: If the big event of the year is on Saturday, for example, drink only tea and water from Tuesday to Friday, but drink these in enormous quantities—five to six liters a day. (For the amount you'll be training, this can't hurt anyway!) Eat according to plan.

Starting Friday at noon, drink nothing at all. Instead, start taking an herbal diuretic, for instance, juniper berries. This will make your body eliminate water like a waterfall—so it wouldn't hurt to have a good book ready in the bathroom. On Friday afternoon you can start eating carbs again, such as rice or gluten-free pasta. This will feed up your muscles and show them to best advantage.

You can start drinking fluids again around noon on Saturday. If you start tossing back drinks on Saturday night, your muscles will start "dancing the samba," as Thomas Wenzl put it.

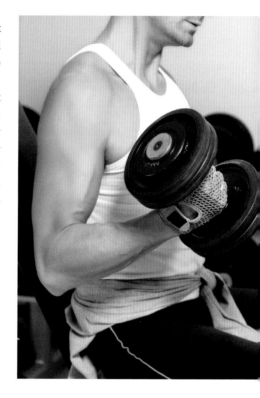

Important Health Warning

During the training period you may experience feelings of dizziness, especially at the start. After all, you are depriving the body of sugar which will confuse it. This deficit is compensated by ingesting more vitamins than usual, so that the unpleasant sensation should subside after a short time.

On the whole, this program also acts as a sensational cleanse for your entire body, as you'll be flushing out all kinds of harmful substances. However, if you do experience any serious discomfort during the two weeks of training, stop training immediately and consult your doctor.

Bon Appétit – The Diet Plan

Even the best training plan will only work properly if you also adjust your diet.

To ensure that you achieve the best results for your figure with our emergency program, Thomas Wenzl has also devised a diet plan that will speed things up even more.

As always, keep in mind that everybody will respond differently to a diet. Food is processed differently, calories are stored differently, and nutrients are converted into energy differently. Which is why I shall dispense with pages and pages of details on the amounts of protein, fat, or whatever. This diet plan is a guideline you can use as an orientation, but you do not have to adhere to it slavishly. Determine what agrees with you personally by experimenting a little!

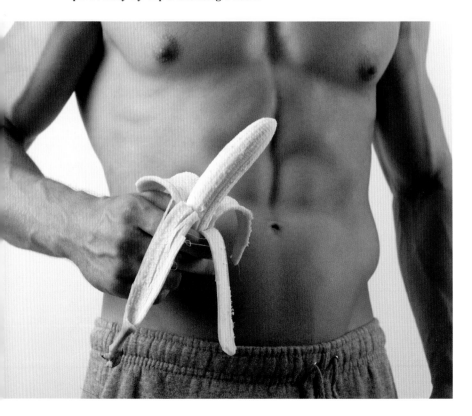

DIET PLAN FOR THE REBEL-WENZL-FOURTEEN-DAY-EMERGENCY-PROGRAM

Breakfast	200 g of sauerkraut, 50 g of crisp bread, 100 g of cucumber
Snack	1 pint of buttermilk, 200 g of pineapple
Noon	300 g of cod, 200 g of broccoli, 200 g of apple
Snack	1 pint of buttermilk, 200 g of banana
Supper	300 g of turkey breast, 200 g of iceberg lettuce
Breakfast	200 g of sauerkraut, 50 g of crisp bread, 100 g of cucumber
Snack	1 pint of buttermilk, 300 g of blueberries
Noon	200 g of beef steak, 200 g of broccoli, 200 g of apple
Snack	200 g of cream cheese, 100 g of cucumber
Supper	300 g of cod, 200 g of iceberg lettuce
Breakfast	200 g of sauerkraut, 100 g of cucumber, 50 g of whole grain bread
Snack	1 pint of buttermilk, 300 g of blueberries
Noon	300 g of turkey breast, 200 g of iceberg lettuce
Snack	200 g of cream cheese, 200 g of cucumber
Supper	200 g of beef steak, 200 g of zucchini
Breakfast	200 g of sauerkraut, 100 g of cucumber, 50 g of whole grain bread
Snack	200 g of cream cheese, 100 g of cucumber
Noon	300 g of calamari, 200 g of broccoli
Snack	200 g of cream cheese, 100 g of cucumber
Supper	300 g of turkey breast, 200 g of asparagus
Breakfast	200 g of sauerkraut, 100 g of cucumber, 50 g of whole grain bread
Snack	200 g of cream cheese, 100 g of cucumber
Noon	300 g of cod, 200 g of asparagus
Snack	200 g of cream cheese, 200 g of cucumber
Supper	300 g of turkey breast, 200 g of iceberg lettuce

Six-Packs for Sex Acts

The fit gay man's ultimate status symbol is probably his six-pack—leaving out the bear fraction, who prefer to present a large hairy ball of lard over their belts as an erotic mating signal.

For the larger part of the male population however, there is no wrist-watch, no car, and no pair of designer jeans that will ever be exhibited and enjoyed quite as much as a sexy set of well-defined abs—if you've got them.

Now there are countless books, DVDs, and well-intentioned articles available in men's magazines with all kinds of top secret tricks on how to get those coveted grooves in your belly. Well, if it's that easy, it's a bit strange that there are still comparatively few guys around with really nice abs. So, it can't be that easy. Nor is it! On the contrary, it can be difficult as hell to build up a six-pack, if nature has not deemed you one of those chosen few for whom it is child's play.

And it's not enough to just work your abs to get a proper six-pack! For people to be able to admire your sexy work of art, you have to have a body fat content of ten percent or less. That's the only way you'll look like a sex god, even in a relaxed position.

Every additional gram of body fat will cover up the small strands of muscle like a thick blanket, destroying all your hard work. So in addition to the proper exercises you will also have to follow a strict diet. In order to really reduce your body fat content, I recommend an extensive diet or a fast. Both of these will help you lose oodles of water and body fat—the dreaded "six-pack-concealers!"

Otherwise the rule is to make sure your diet is low in carbohydrates. A recent study has shown that overweight men lose up to three times as much fat from the middle of their bodies by cutting out carbs than by a low-fat diet! The following foods should, among others, definitely be avoided, if you want to let other people see the beautiful trained muscles dance underneath your skin:

Very Bad:
- bread, especially white bread
- rice
- potatoes
- sugar
- white pasta
- fast food / pizza
- saturated fats
- carbonated sodas
- isoglucose or corn syrup (just check the ingredient list—you'll be surprised at all the stuff you'll find there)

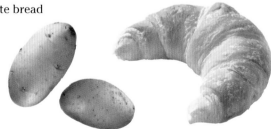

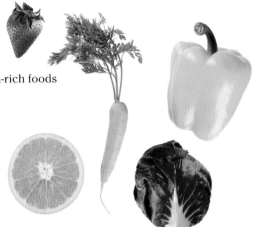

Very Good:

- chicken
- fish and other protein-rich foods
- lean meat
- fruit and vegetables
- nuts
- oats
- cottage cheese
- low-fat curds
- olive oil
- whole grain bread

OK, and now it's time for the bitter truth: Not every man has a nice six-pack lying dormant under his skin. The abdominal muscles consist of different muscle groups that are positioned differently in every man. Your straight muscles may well be positioned off-center instead of lying straight across your abdomen. Your oblique abs may also be positioned higher up than you would like—depending on how Mother Nature created you, even a view of your midriff unobscured by rolls of fat may still not present the right look. If you aren't built that way naturally, even the toughest training won't help. But let's be honest here, it's not all about the abs. The right training will transform your entire body for the better. That way, it's a complete and delicious package you'll be delivering, not just a run-of-the-mill presentation six-pack. As I don't want to totally destroy your illusions about the six-pack myth, here are a few basic rules:

Hot Abs 1

Watch Your Breathing!
Never hold your breath. Breathe in as you tense your abs and breathe out when you relax them.

Hot Abs 2

Watch Your Speed!
The more slowly you perform an exercise, the stronger the effect. You're not trying to beat any speed records, but should rather be concentrating on each exercise. If an exercise is too easy, you can, of course, just add more weight. But consult your trainer first.

Hot Abs 3

Watch Your Strength!

If you feel you can't go on, then continue with the exercise anyway, until you simply have to stop. Overcome your inner lazy bones! You're stronger than you think you are. It takes extreme discipline (and really sore muscles) to achieve a really hot six-pack. In order for your muscles to grow, the last painful repetitions are the most important.

Hot Abs 4

Watch Your Preparation!

Always warm up properly before training your abs. At least twenty minutes of endurance training are reasonable. The body doesn't even start burning up fat deposits before that time. Look at it as killing two birds with one stone: on the one hand, you're preparing your muscles for exertion and minimizing the risk of injury. On the other, you're burning up your dreaded body fat. Try jumping rope—there is hardly anything more effective, and you won't be tempted to cheat, as frequently occurs when cycling. It also trains the entire body. Do all this on an empty stomach and there will nothing left standing between you and the ten percent body fat of your dreams!

Hot Abs 5

Watch Your Posture!

Your lower back should always be lying flat on a mat and not raised during the workout—unless, of course, this is part of the exercise. Keep your pelvis pressed towards your navel—that way you'll stay in the right position automatically. To prevent yourself from throwing your head up, it's best to keep your hands around your ears rather than at the back of your neck. Keep your gaze fixed towards the ceiling and make sure there is a hand's breadth between your chin and your chest. Concentrate on doing the exercise! You should feel the movement in your abs. Listen to your body and try to feel every single muscle on its own.

Hot Abs 6

Watch the Variety!

Muscles are a bit like children with ADHD—they need a lot of variety. Routines will only make them switch off and work with just a fraction of the strength available—with weaker results to match. So switch up the exercises from workout to workout. You can also add variations within the workout: train first the lower abs, then the obliques, and then the upper abs. Focus on a different muscle group every day!

Hot Abs 7

Watch Your Back!
Don't neglect your back, otherwise the balance between your abdominal muscles and your back muscles will be lost. Both muscle groups are directly dependent on one another.

Hot Abs 8

Take A Reality Check!
Please remember: everyone responds differently to exercise. Some people will respond immediately to certain exercises and others will have to toil endlessly for only half the results. It is important to pay attention to your body's signals: which exercises work for me, which don't, where can I see results, where can't I see any?
Don't throw in the towel right away. It's well worth the effort, as a yummy six-pack is a real sex magnet!

Hot Abs 9

Watch Your Enjoyment!
No matter how tough the training, if you don't enjoy it, you will never be satisfied with the results. Try and make your workouts as enjoyable as possible—even if it does sometimes seem hard.

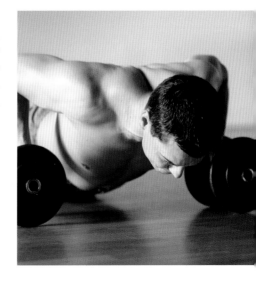

How Often Should You Train?

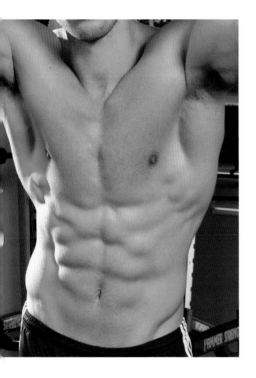

During the first couple of weeks you should perform an intense abs workout every two days. Once you start feeling yourself getting stronger, increase the amount to once a day. Overtraining is highly unlikely, as abdominals take a shorter time to regenerate than other muscles. But do give yourself a few days off every four weeks at the latest, so that you're not completely exhausted and irritable from training.

Do twenty to twenty-five repeats per exercise. That doesn't sound like much, but if you perform the exercise slowly and consciously, you'll easily reach your pain threshold. The trick is not to do more repeats but rather to perform a single exercise more slowly. Because if you do more than twenty-five repeats, you're actually training for endurance rather than strength. So, make every exercise more difficult and make your muscles contract harder, so that you really can *do* only twenty repeats.

Let's Go — The Exercises!

On the following pages, Thomas and I will be presenting our abs training program. If you really take this program to heart, I guarantee you'll be good step closer to the six-pack of your dreams.

To facilitate understanding, the following thirteen exercises have been illustrated by photos of Thomas. Make sure you perform these exercises exactly as we describe them.

Bicycle Crunches

The top exercise for your abs!
That was the result of an American study on the most popular exercises and their effects. The Bicycle Crunch was shown to be the most effective exercise of them all for successfully building up a six-pack. Sadly, it is also one of the hardest, and is therefore only recommended for more advanced training, once you have already built up some basic strength in your abs.

• To do the Bicycle Crunch, lie on your back, your hands behind your ears, elbows out to the sides. Then pull your right knee towards your chest while at the same time pulling your left elbow towards the same knee.

• Then extend your right leg again and, in a fluid motion, pull your left knee to your right elbow.

• Always do this exercise in a slow and concentrated manner. Keep your lower back flat on the floor at all times!

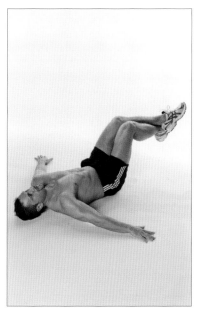

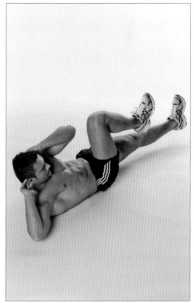

Hardcore Bicycle Crunches

The standard Bicycle Crunch isn't enough for you?
• Lie on your back, your arms out to the sides.
• Then raise your upper body while pulling your right leg towards your chest. Push forwards with your hands from either side, as if you were pressing against an invisible wall. Your left leg should be stretched out just above the floor. Hold for five seconds.
• Then slowly extend your leg again and pull your arms back into the starting position.
• Repeat with the left leg—and that's one repeat.
• Do 25 repeats! (If you can do this easily, you probably already have a very nice six-pack. Photographic evidence should be sent to svenrebel@web.de!)

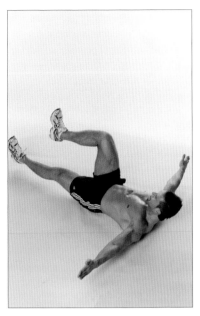

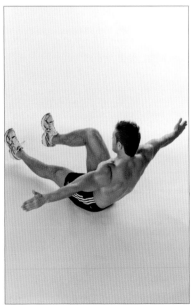

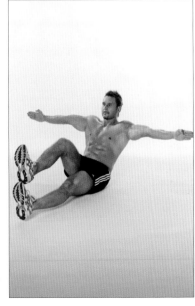

Crunches

• Lie on the floor, resting your feet on a chair, so that your legs form a 90° angle. (For the advanced, dispense with the chair and hold your feet up in the air.)
• Stretch your arms forward and then your head, slowly, then raise your neck and shoulders from the ground and curl them under—as if you were trying to touch your chest with your chin.
• You should be pulling your upper body up with your abs, try and feel it. Your lower back should stay flat on the ground.
• Pull your upper body towards your chest as far as you can, hold for five seconds and then slower lower yourself down again.

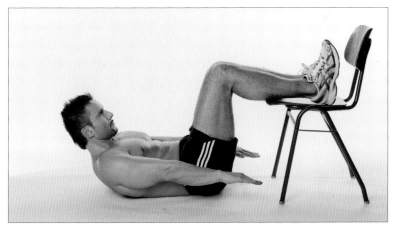

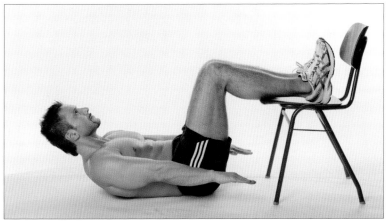

The Plank

Is tougher than it sounds!
• Lie on your front, supporting your weight on your elbows, which should be parallel to your shoulders. Your upper body will automatically be hanging in mid-air as if your were going to do a push-up.
• Your lower body should be resting on your knees and toes so that your heels point upwards and are parallel.
• Then extend your knees, tensing your body so that it is balanced on your elbows and toes.
• Your body should form a straight line. So, don't push your hips up or let them hang down. I recommend using a mirror or getting a partner to check for you. It should look as if you had a stick going down from your head to your feet.
• Hold this position for as long as possible. Your abs and all your other muscles should be flexed.
• Don't forget to breathe evenly the entire time; something you can easily forget during this exercise.

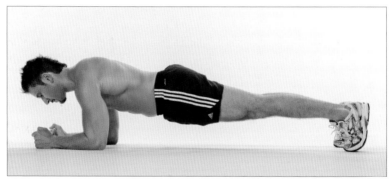

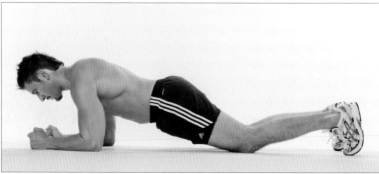

Hip Raises

Work the lower abs
• Lie on your back, knees bent and arms extended to either side.
• Then raise your legs to form a right angle between your hips and your thighs.
• Stretch your legs straight up and cross your feet.
• Then slowly roll your butt up from the floor towards the ceiling as far as you can. Imagine you're trying to touch the ceiling with your toes.
• Then slowly lower your hips without lowering your behind all the way. In a fluid motion, push your hips up again. If this exercise is too hard for you, support your spine by sliding your hands underneath your butt.

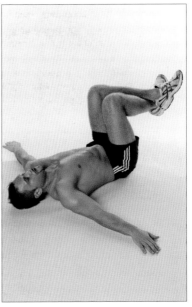

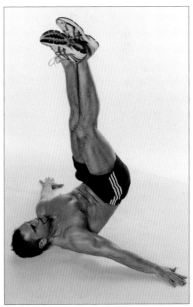

Reverse Crunches

• Lie on your back with your head slightly raised.
• Then raise your bent legs and slowly pull them towards your chest, raising your hips.
• Hold briefly.
• Slowly lower your legs again, but don't put them down all the way. Instead hold them briefly just above the ground and then pull them towards your chest again.

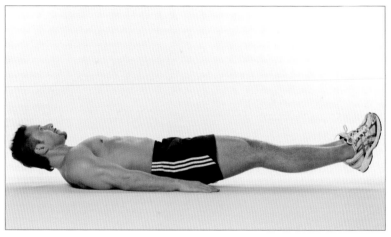

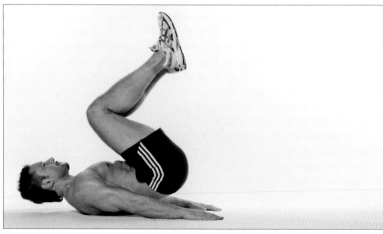

The L

This incredibly effective exercise also works the lower abs. You will need two push-up stands or a bar.

• Sit down straight, both legs extended. Place your hands on the stands and push up, raising your butt off the ground.

• Tense your legs so that they are also raised off the ground and hold in a right angle to your upper body.

• The higher you hold your legs, the harder and the more effective the exercise. Your goal is to raise and hold your legs so high that the L becomes a V.

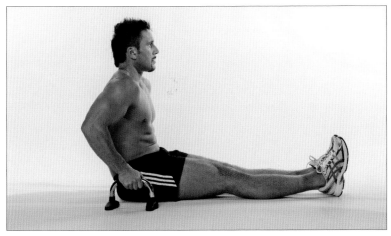

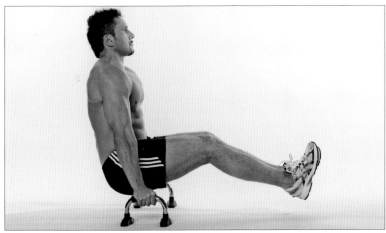

Extended Crunches

• Lie on your back, hands behind the back of your neck and elbows to the sides.
• Stretch your legs, raising them slightly so that they are held flat over the ground. Press into the ground with your hips and cross your feet.
• Then slowly raise your head and shoulders about twelve inches above the ground. Hold briefly and lower again. The pull should come from your abs—do not pull at your head with your arms.

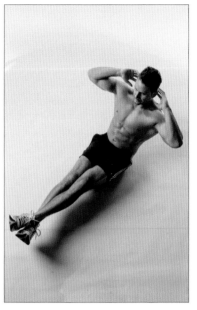

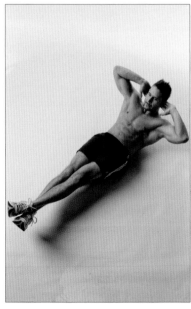

Oblique Crunches

Work the oblique abs
• Lie on your side with your legs bent at a 90° angle, so that your knees are in front of your hips.
• Twist your head and shoulders back so that your shoulder blades and the back of your head lie flat on the floor.
• The use your abs to pull your upper body straight up—as far as possible. Slowly and carefully, lower it again. Repeat twenty-five times.
• Then do the same with your knees on the other side of your body.

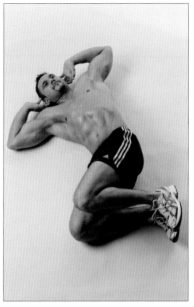

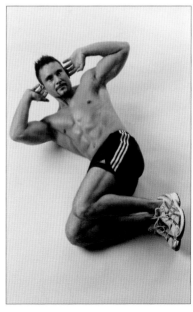

Side Bridge

Another good exercise for the oblique abs
• Lie stretched out on your right side, supporting your upper body on your left elbow.
• Then tense your body and raise your hips up off the ground until you're only supported by your right elbow and right foot.
• Your body should form a straight line from your head to your foot.
• Hold this position for thirty seconds, then slowly lower your body back down. Do twenty-five repeats on one side.
• Repeat the entire exercise on your left side.

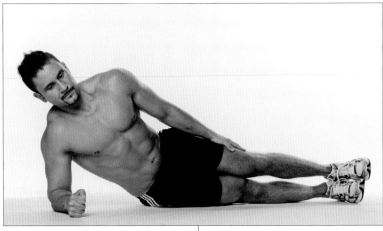

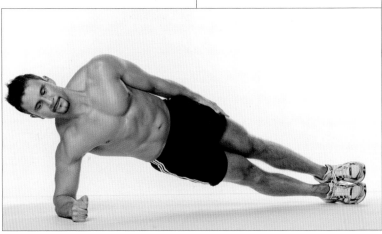

The Dog

A good beginner's exercise
• Support yourself with your hands and knees on the floor.
• Tense your abs and raise your knees slightly off the ground so that your weight is supported by your hands and toes.
• Then bend your right leg slightly, raising your right foot off the ground. Now you should be supported only by your hands and your left foot.
• Hold the position for thirty seconds. The easier this exercise is for you, the longer you should hold it.
• Lower your right foot again and repeat with your left foot.

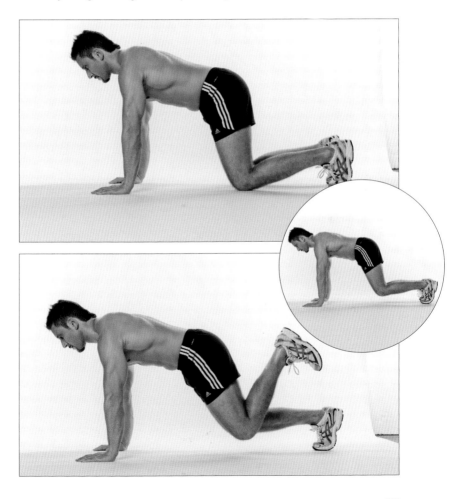

Kicks

A more advanced exercise, as you will need good body tension to perform this workout
• Lie on your back, arms crossed over your chest, legs extended.
• Raise your legs slightly so that your feet are floating just above the ground.
• Pull your left leg towards your chest and then kick forwards hard without your feet touching the floor. Your lower back should be firmly pressed to the floor.
• Repeat with the left leg!

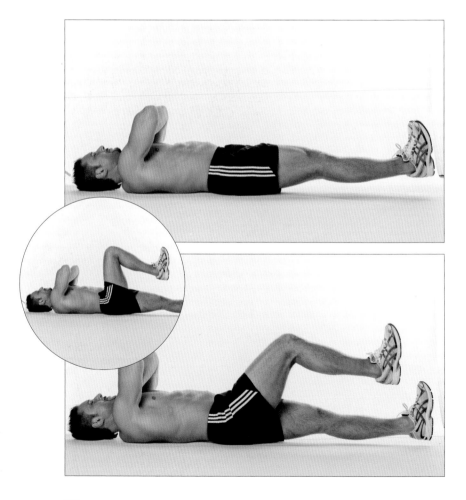

The Boat

Another difficult exercise which should only be attempted once you are strong enough
• Lie on your back, your arms stretched out flat on the floor behind your head, your body tensed.
• Raise your outstretched arms and legs about eight inches off the floor, keeping your body taut—stiffen it up!
• Then slowly rock back and forth twenty-five times, like a boat on the water.

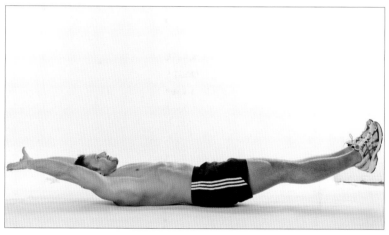

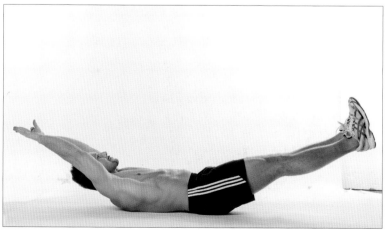

The Terrible Truth

As I have said, this program will take you a step further towards the six-pack of your dreams, but you must realize that it can be really tough going, depending on how your body responds to training. Everyone should first consider whether it's really worth the effort.

I have managed to achieve a really hot six-pack once in my life—and there is not a trace of it left today. If you don't keep it up, even the best-defined abs will soon sink back into oblivion. For me personally, the effort was simply too great, as sadly I am of the physical type that quickly builds up muscle which is nonetheless very hard to define. But it's just that definition that you need for a proper six-pack. And once your abs become a full-time job, it stops being fun. Admittedly, I do envy those guys who are natural athletes and who can present a perfect six-pack with comparatively little effort. But hey, there are plenty of people out there who prefer a more heavyset kind of guy. At least I know it's possible if I really want to do it. And if I can do it, it shouldn't be that hard for you!

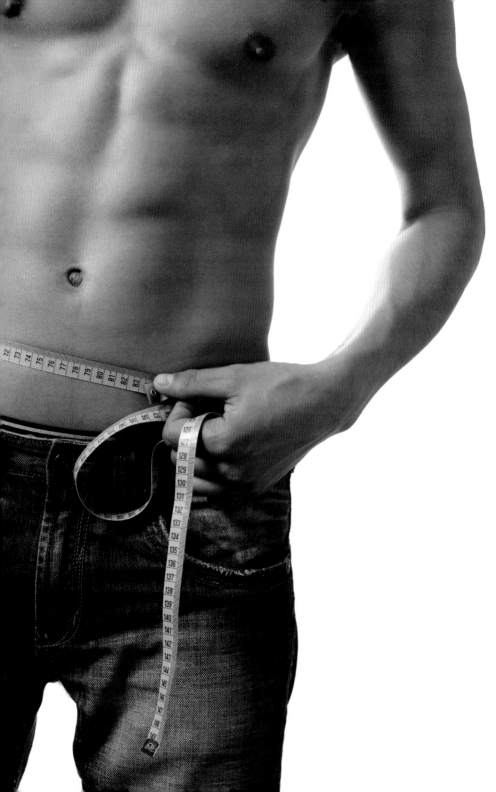

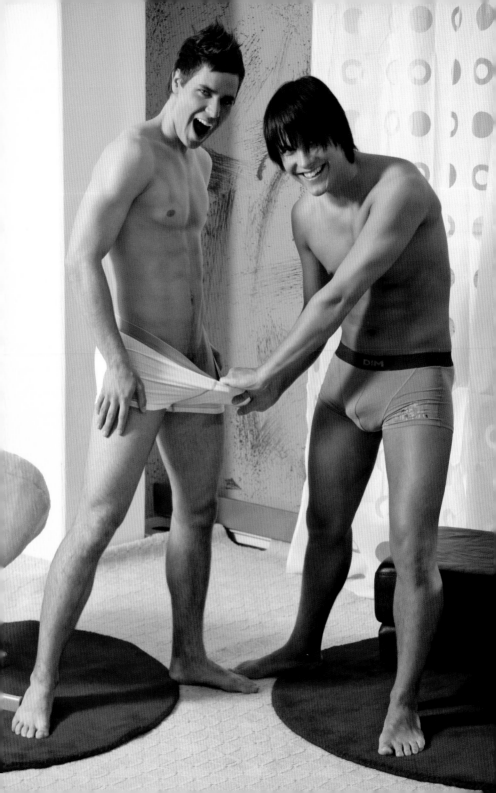

Sex II

As you can never know too much about the best thing in the world, here are some more wonderfully useful and ridiculous facts about sex.

My Hero

The champion of the long jizz is an Italian engineer who can ejaculate an amazing twenty-one yards, down to the last inch. However, this incredible gift is not due to his superior potency but rather to a deformation of his pelvic muscles. To protect him from sexual harassment I will not be publishing his name here.

Libido

In an official study, forty-five percent of the men asked admitted to wanting more sex in their love lives. Perhaps they should try having sex without love—that's fun, too!

A Gem

For the medical profession, a small penis is one under an inch in length—they call it a micropenis! It is doubtful whether this will make the guys out there who are just over an inch feel any better.

Handiwork

Most men—that is about twenty-three percent of those able to masturbate—do it once every two days. To balance it out, nine percent jerk off twice a day.

Measuring Up

To remove all doubts as to the acceptability of your penis size: The average penis is 3.5 to 3.7 inches when soft. When erect, it grows to measure between 5 and 5.7 inches. Funnily enough, most of the guys on gay Web sites claim to be way above average.

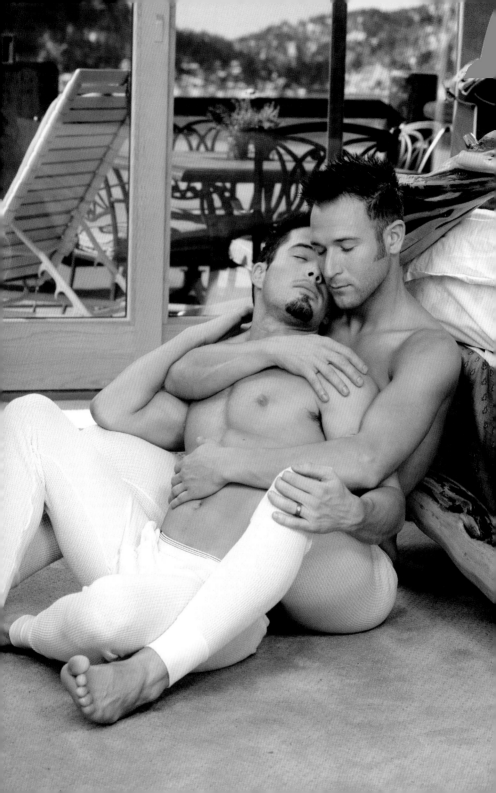

Interpersonal Skills

As much as I appreciate all the wonderful new opportunities the Inter-net has bestowed upon us, there is one thing I will never forgive the World Wide Web for: Nobody knows how to flirt properly these days! While getting to know a guy online at any time of the day or night is no trouble at all, the younger set in particular are finding it more and more difficult to make a move on another man on the street, in a café, or in any other public place. If you grow up with the certainty of getting into a willing partner's pants with just a few clicks, you will one day come to the painful realization that lines like "and what are you into?" or "show me your dick" rarely have much success when uttered at the supermarket checkout. This creates a vicious circle: Ignorance and insecurity mean that nobody is brave enough to flirt in public anymore. And so guys look for contacts online, and more and more of them forget how much more exciting it is to meet nice guys in real life.

In the same way, the fine art of elegantly ending a relationship/affair is dying out. Admittedly, it's never very nice, but in real life it is a bit more complicated than just blocking the former object of your desire online. Whether these drastic methods of ending a relationship are a blessing or a curse is up for debate. But they certainly never convey mutual respect. For there is one thing I would like to stress: If you at any point in time have had strong feelings, perhaps even love, for a guy and then you just unceremoniously dump him, how much value are you ascribing to your former feelings? And how much will they be worth in the future? Won't your feelings become increasingly trivial and arbitrary?

But enough of these philosophical questions. Of course, one thing is clear: If the guy you love hurts you, lies to you, or cheats on you, then of course he's fired the first shot and you have every right to counter with whatever weapon you've got.

In any case, it is time to take up arms against the current trend of a virtual "click-and-fuck" society: boys, get yourselves outside! Flirt as you've never flirted before, on the streets, in the office, at the movies, and at the IRS.

Not only will you increase the likelihood of finding the man of your dreams, a bit of flirting will improve the atmosphere in every city. And that benefits all of us. Besides, meeting a new person can be incredibly exciting if you're not immediately presented with a list of all his personal and sexual preferences on his profile page, and aren't forced to gauge the complicated mechanism of a man according to these couple of qualities. Flirting and dating increases your tolerance threshold and your curiosity, and makes you want to try out something new. If you really believe you're only a bottom, you'll never meet another bottom man online. But if you meet a guy in a café, without knowing anything about him and fall head over heels in love with him, you might just realize that applying every trick in the book to his hot body might not be such a bad thing after all.

It is time to turn off your computer and turn your gaze back to the men in the real world outside. There are any number of hot and exciting adventures waiting for you out there. To make the step outside a little easier for you, here's a flirting, dating, and breaking up 101.

Flirt with Me!

Flirting works on five levels: Whenever two people meet, a program starts up inside each of them, automatically checking off the following points: What does he look like, what does he sound like, what does he smell like, what does he feel like, and what does he taste like. A few seconds are enough for our unconscious mind to take in the tiniest pieces of information relayed by all our sensory organs. So, we instantly form a complete impression, resulting in liking, indifference, or rejection. There is much I could write about this topic, for it is fascinating how many signals we send out to other people—and, of course, receive from them—without being conscious of the fact.

That's why it's important to be aware that we have to make an effort on a number of levels if we want to ignite a flaming inferno of lust in another man.

The following pages will discuss what you should pay attention to when flirting:

Your Looks

Sure, looks are important, but they aren't everything. Most people are familiar with the situation where you think you're meeting a really hot guy, but the very first word that comes out of his mouth dispels every trace of the fascination he held for us. Sometimes an affected laugh, an odd way of walking, or ears that stick out are enough. It's generally the small things you start to hate after a while. But fortunately, looks are a matter of taste, and so it's not only supermodels who will find a partner but maybe also people who are not good-looking, but are cute, sexy, or simply amazingly charming and intelligent instead.

There are any number of chapters in this book on how to optimize your looks. That way, even the ugliest duckling has a good chance of becoming a halfway acceptable swan. It's always worth leaving a good impression whenever you go out in public, looking well-groomed and smelling nice, for you never know if Mr. Right will be just around the corner. Besides which, you'll simply feel better and look more confident if you know you're looking sharp. So, always make sure there's no food stuck between your teeth, that your breath and your underpants are fresh as a daisy, that your T-shirt doesn't have a brownish yellow stain on it and that your armpits aren't exuding a reminder of your last workout.

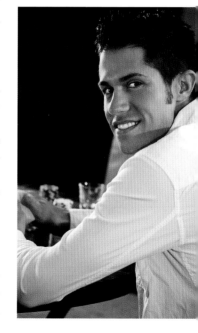

The Location

You can basically flirt anywhere, although you might want to avoid making any blatant passes at a Westboro Baptist Church meeting.

Supposedly the top flirting location is the Laundromat. Closely followed by the food department of a fancy department store, perhaps because both places have an above average number of single customers.

But it would still be silly to trundle back and forth between the dairy aisle, the noodles, and the dryers in the hopes of bumping into your next partner. It's definitely a good idea to try places where other gay men hang out. So, try the more expensive boutiques in your neighborhood, the movie theater (when they're playing something with Meryl Streep or Sarah Jessica Parker), or simply the better known gay cafés in town. (You can also find great hordes of gay men in the park, but they are generally there to fuck rather than talk.)

The best strategy is to keep your eyes open everywhere and at all times and just toss out a nice friendly smile if you see anyone you like—you'll be surprised at how much can grow from such a small gesture.

By the way, if you go to a club, make sure you're visible. If you stand in a corner behind the door all night, it won't be surprising if no one flirts with you. An old friend told me once: "The person dancing in the middle of the dance floor is always desirable." And it's true. Always place yourself strategically so that everyone can see you. For how is the man of your dreams supposed to find you if he can't see you anywhere? The more people see you, the greater the chance that one of them will be someone whose dream guy you are.

Confidence

Sure, a shy glance can be a real heartbreaker. But usually, a bashful and wallflower-like demeanor will mean no one will even notice you. That's why it is important to give a confident impression so the object of your desires will actually notice you. Remember: a man who acts confident is almost always a sex magnet!

If an impressive bearing is difficult for you, here's a very good exercise: when you wake up in the morning, stay in bed for another couple of minutes and think about what it would be like to be the most irresistible man in the world. What would it be like if all the great guys you're into were into you as well? Imagine how that might feel. Then try and recreate this sensation for yourself all day long. Just behave as if your wish had come true. Play the game, be an actor! It doesn't matter if it makes you feel weird, just do it! I guarantee you'll be surprised at how quickly you'll experience a changed reaction in the people around you—a positive one. Plan on doing this at least once a week, a day to let yourself hit the love jackpot!

In the long run, it can help to take up sports or register for an ego-training class or autogenic training—all of these will boost your confidence.

Of course, none of this will work if you are pathologically shy and have serious mental health issues. In that case, seeing a therapist is the only thing that will help. But that's fine, too, as long as it gets you closer to your life goals and makes you happier.

Alcohol

Alcohol does loosen your inhibitions and make you think you're flirting more freely, but you end up doing this with a lot less success than when sober. Because who's into drunk, inanely grinning machos spouting one dumb pick-up line after the next? While you're drunk, you may see yourself as a smooth seducer, but others probably see you as an embarrassment. So, never drink more than one or two glasses of Dutch courage. This almost always goes badly, as alcohol makes thinking and speaking more difficult as well as impairing your concentration. Sober is just a lot nicer!

Your Voice

I'm not joking! Men with deep voices are seen as more attractive and desirable. It makes sense, doesn't it? What's the use of a beautifully trained body, if a squeaky voice starts to mumble obscenities from it? There goes that buzz! As flirting is all about getting the whole package right, just try to make a habit of speaking in a slightly deeper voice than usual. Nothing too conspicuous or unnatural, so as to sound ridiculous, but just using a little more air from your lungs and speaking each word more slowly and consciously in a lowered voice. You'll get used to it after a while and then you'll see that just a couple of words spoken at the right pitch can charm the pants off a really hot guy. If your voice is generally on the squeaky end of the spectrum, register for a voice training class. That will help a lot.

Eye Contact

Of course, the key to successful flirting is making the right eye contact. Research has shown that in our culture, if you look firmly into someone's eyes for more than three seconds, they will see it as an invitation to sex—perhaps that's the reason why straight men get so aggressive if you look at them for too long, as they are all too familiar with the dirty thoughts in our primitive hunter brains, which are always on the lookout for prey. So, never underestimate the power of nonverbal communication through the eyes!

Once you've established eye contact, a confident gaze may get you closer to your goal more quickly, but a shy gaze can also work wonders.

Revealing weakness can often leave a pleasant, likable impression. Mind you, your gaze can be shy, but not the rest of your body language. That will come across as uptight and even repellant—the same way a sickly appearance rarely sends out erotic signals—that's evolution at work.

Once you've made eye contact with another guy, the following signals will give a clear indication of your interest: smiling, blinking, nodding slightly, leaning your head to one side, fixing your clothes, or raising an eyebrow.

You can make your intentions clear to even the most oblivious person by frequently touching the object of your desire accidentally on purpose. But of course, that no longer falls under the heading "Eye Contact."

The Time Factor

Be quick! If you like a guy, respond right away! Tests have shown that thirty seconds after the object of your flirtation has signaled his approval, your chances of reaching the next level will rapidly decrease. So, if he smiles at you, smile back right away! Look deep into his eyes—be clear about your intentions! Even if he looks away, stay on the ball! This is typical of the flirting game, it's simply part of it. The best thing is to speak to him relatively soon after receiving a few unambiguous positive signals. Don't be too impatient, you'll only ruin your chances.

It's enough to walk up to him and say, "Hi, I'm ...!" Generally you can start a conversation from there. Otherwise, you can go ahead and be more direct: "I think you're interesting. Would you like to meet up with me some time?"

Do not memorize any dumb pick-up lines and do not try to be too original. Unless you're a professional actor, a "witty" line will always fall flat. Be yourself! If you're always witty, be witty when you flirt. If you're not a barrel of laughs, why should you be one at this delicate moment in time?

Don't be afraid of being turned down. What's the worst that can happen? If you approach someone nicely, the answer—even if it's negative—will be nice as well. But there's nothing wrong with being turned down. Not everyone has to like you. Think of all the people you don't want to get to know yourself. Maybe they're all really nice, they're just not your type. So, go for it! If you flirt with a guy, there's at least a fifty percent chance of it working out. If you do nothing, there's a one hundred percent chance of being annoyed with yourself later on.

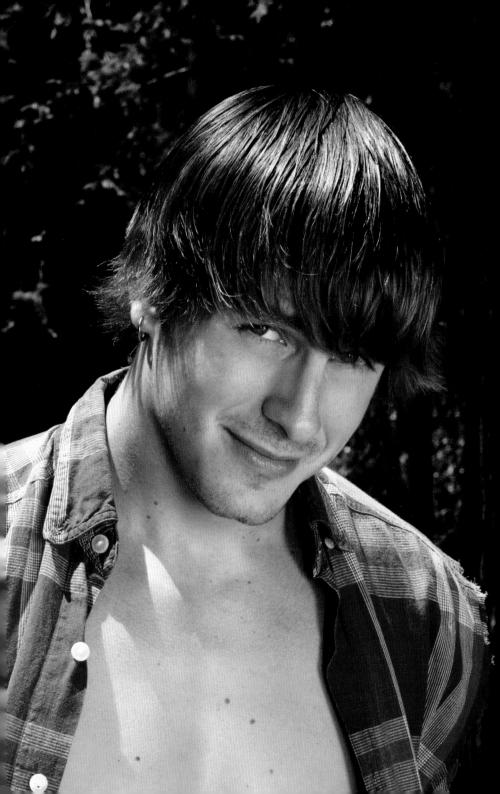

But don't be pushy. "No!" means no! No matter how hard you try, you'll only make it worse. So, accept the rebuff. The next guy is just around the corner.

By the way, for all of you who can't be bothered to speak to another man because you think, "If he wants me, he'll come over": Think about this for a couple of minutes! What if everyone thought the same way? And who do you think you are to be so arrogant? The Queen of England? No? Then pull yourself together and don't behave that way to the people around you!

The Conversation

Once you've spoken to the guy who sets your stomach on fire and you've hesitantly embarked on a conversation, stay on the ball—but be careful. One false or rash statement, and all your hard worked-for prospects will disappear. A few tactics can help in carrying on a conversation, such as: Stay away from the yes-or-no questions. Otherwise the conversation will quickly founder. Ask open questions that require lengthier answers.

Which means, avoid questions like: "Do you like music/movies/the theater?" They will get you a bare "yes" or "no" if you're unlucky, and then you'll have to cast out a new verbal line to get the conversation going properly.

This is important: Be interested in the other man's answers. Silence can really be golden when you're meeting new people. A good listener is easily likable. From time to time, of course, you should relate a bit about yourself so that the conversation doesn't get too impersonal and one-sided. But try to get the guy across from you to open up. Ask questions like: "What do you think about …?" or "Where are you from?" or "What are your experiences with …?" In general, good conversational questions begin with who, where, what, how, and why.

Make sure your questions aren't too intimate. At all costs, avoid topics that could lead to arguments or debate, such as religion, disease, or politics. At no point should you ask him about his exes, nor should you describe your plans for the future with this new acquaintance.

Let your charm do the rest, even if you don't think you have any—if you're excited and interested in the guy, you will most certainly be charming. Be polite and pay him the occasional compliment.

Humor is another important aspect. If you can make him laugh, that's a guaranteed path to his pants, as well as heart. But please don't try too hard to be funny—you are not a stand-up comedian at work.

Be interesting about everything you say about yourself. Of course you shouldn't tell lies, but put yourself in a good light, accentuate the positive—in short: Sell yourself! After all, you are the best catch for miles around, aren't you? Just consider whether the hobby you are so passionate about, be it bird watching, collecting spoons or macramé, is really that interesting to someone else. Sometimes it's better to keep a lid on the leisure activities you're really fanatical about.

Patience
Be Patient! Very Patient!

Just because you're into this guy and are itching to get your sticky paws on him doesn't mean he feels the same about you. Perhaps he needs a bit more time or perhaps he'd just like to get to know you better. Don't be pushy or overpowering.

For lasting success, you'll need time and plenty of patience!

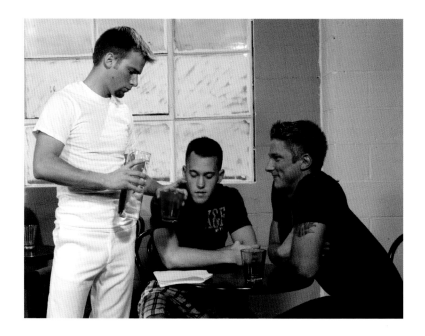

Practice Makes Perfect

Get out there and practice your flirting technique. Not just on guys you really like, because they might make you nervous and you'll ruin everything. Try flirting with a few guys you like just a little. For one thing, it's a great way of honing your skills which will make you more confident where it matters and at the same time you'll brighten up the day for all the men you flirt with, making a city of happy homos.

Turning Down an Advance

Being on the receiving end of flirtations and pick-up lines feels fantastic and is one of the greatest compliments you can get. Unfortunately, some guys don't get that they don't stand a chance of hearing anything but a nice "No thanks!" Most likely drunk, they continue to try and pick you up and generally get on your nerves. The only thing that can help is a witty put-down at the right moment, preferably launched at him in front of his friends—sometimes you have to get tough!

Here are a couple of lines to keep up your sleeve for the appropriate time:

Emergency Lines For a Quick Put-Down

TOP TEN QUICK PUT-DOWN

10 Hey, if I wanted to kill myself, I'd climb your ego and jump to your IQ.

9 It looks like your face caught on fire and someone tried to put it out with a hammer.

8 Why don't you come back when you have less time?

7 You're looking for a guy with a sense of humor? Well, that's all you can hold out for!

6 Say, were your parents into anal? 'Cause you look really shitty!

5 Has anyone ever told you you look really sexy? No? Well, they won't!

4 Do you want to lose ten pounds of ugly fat? Cut off your head!

3 Sit on the ground, it's used to dirt!

2 Your birth certificate is an apology letter from the condom factory.

My all-time favorite put-down is dedicated to all those women who simply won't accept that you're gay and not remotely interested in them, and who just keep getting on your nerves. The ultimate line that will immediately offend every girl and get her off your back is this one:

1 "Say, girlfriend, would you buy shoes if you had no feet? No? Then why did you buy a bra?" That should do it. She'll leave you in peace and spend the rest of the evening crying in the toilets. The funny thing is, this line works just as well on women with enormous boobs. Don't ask me why, but I tried it and it worked!

Five Tips for Your First (Real) Date

Let's say you've climbed the first hurdle and made a date with your dream guy. There are still a couple of things you need to pay attention to in order to have a successful date.

If you're just meeting for sex, this chapter won't be of much interest to you. But—and this is just a suggestion here—try a proper date the next time, not just a hookup. It's worth it!

Be Generous!

If you're really into this guy, pay the bill—for the entire evening. Forget all that nonsense about splitting the check. Show your date you're serious, that you're a man of grace and decorum, and that you respect him enough to fork over some cash. Of course, you should make sure you can actually afford your chosen location first. And do make sure you have enough cash on you. There's nothing more embarrassing than offering to pay and then having to ask your date to lend you money.

Choose the Right Location!

As I mentioned above, you should, of course, choose a location that's within your means. But try and come up with something special. The movies are a terrible choice—how are you going to get to know each other if you hardly exchange a word for half the evening. Besides, choosing the right film can lead to arguments, which will nip your burgeoning relationship in the bud. Even if you see yourself as a cineast, reading three hours of subtitles about the misery of a twelve-year-old Croatian girl following a miscarriage is not for everyone.

If you're really strapped for cash, improvise. A picnic at your local park, a cool museum, or even dinner at your place—as long as your apartment is presentable, meaning clean and tidy and not smelling of old kitty litter.

"Less is more" is always a good rule for a first date. Don't use up all your ideas right away—keep a few more up your sleeve for the next date—after all, you want to up the ante, don't you?

Be Punctual!

Do whatever you have to do to be on time! Be at the arranged place punctually at the arranged time—and absolutely do not cancel at the last minute just because you don't feel like it. You'll regret it when you try to arrange a second date.

Respect!

Respect the other man's opinions. No matter what the subject is. Dates are for getting to know one another, not for converting the other person to your personal world view. And don't forget: show an interest in what the other man tells you. Don't just talk about yourself. Be sincerely interested!

Make a Good Impression!

Turn up for your date looking good. Meaning, be clean and properly groomed. Just make a good impression—unless, of course, you're meeting a guy who's into grungy, smelly types. But then you probably wouldn't be going on a proper date, instead you'd just meet in some grubby corner and behave like trash.

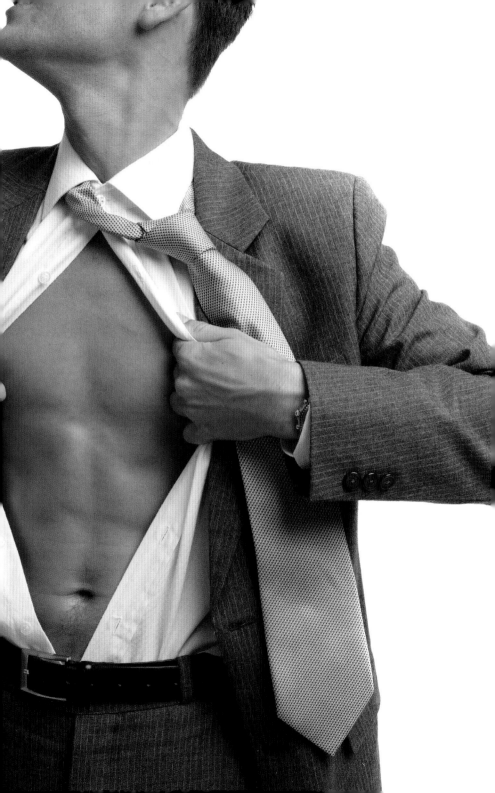

Stay on the Ball!

At the end of a nice date, ask politely whether you can see him again. No matter how desperate you are, don't invite him home with you or go to his place.

Does this make me sound old-fashioned? Sure! But this method will lead you directly into the heart of a man with serious intentions, as you'll be behaving differently from pretty much everyone else. The object of your desire will feel adored rather than like a sex-object—and that can lead to much more. Besides, denying yourself sex on the first night is a great way of testing whether your date is really interested in you. If he's only into sex, then he'll come up with a thousand reasons to turn down another date with you. That way, at least you'll know where you stand!

P.S. Of course, if you just want to fuck, these tips don't count. Just tell him right off and save yourself the effort!

Cocktails – Cool Drinks for a Hot Date

Shaken or stirred—whenever a hot little number comes to your place for the first time, you can always impress him by smoothly offering him a suitable cocktail. While you're mixing drinks, it's easy to strike up a conversation and you can avoid awkward gaps in the conversation that way. With just a little skillful maneuvering, you can also get a bit closer to your love interest; instead of awkwardly perching next to him, you can either involve him in preparing the drinks or accidentally touch him a couple of times to let him know your intentions. Remember: passionate action is always better than passiveness.

But good cocktails aren't just great for a hot date, you can impress pretty much any crowd by casually shaking up a drink at the right moment. And even if you're just sitting around at home, alone and depressed, a good strong alcoholic mix can always provide a bit of dignity and class.

Now, there are simply billions of different cocktails: they can be sweet and creamy, colorful but strong, a liqueur mix, frozen or hot. There are short drinks and long drinks, before- and after-dinner drinks—the more you try and keep up in the world of cocktails, the more impossible it seems. But there are a few classics that have established themselves over the years and are always a safe bet. Apart from the mixture in your glass, the decoration is also an important part of every drink's image—an olive, for instance, is a wonderfully manly addition to your martini glass, while a medium-sized fruit basket perched on the edge of a glass of fruit punch is anathema to every gender, and should only be seen in the hands of dumb teenagers who don't know any better. As a rule, you should leave out the little umbrellas and similar folderol—otherwise your date might think you're either insane or a holiday cruise director on the run.

For you, the rule is: Always mix a man's cocktail. Women prefer other drinks in general. Be careful with sweet cocktails as well. These generally

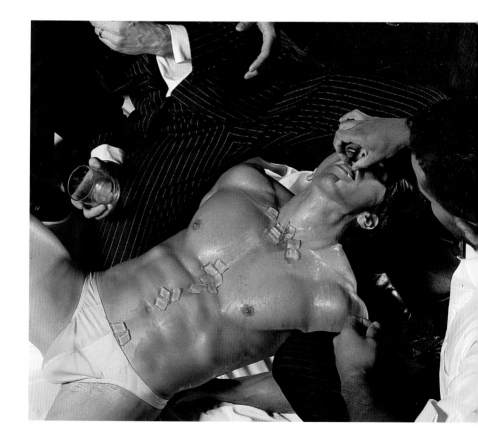

contain far too many sugary, creamy ingredients. If you drink one of these potions, your stomach will swell up as if you'd eaten a five-course meal at a fast food stand and you can forget about dancing the mattress jig for the rest of the evening. These creamy drinks will not only make you uncomfortably full, the sugar will gum up every willing orifice. Instead, check out my list of the top six men's cocktails for a hot date:

TOP SIX COCKTAILS

6 The Classic: Long Island Ice Tea
It looks harmless, but it's strong enough to force many a man to his knees. The secret lies in the huge amounts of hard spirits that form the basis of this drink—none of them ice tea! The finished product just looks that way. You can never go wrong with a Long Island Ice Tea. On the contrary—if you can mix a Long Island Ice Tea, you'll be beloved by everyone, from the bitchiest mother-in-law to the hottest guy in town. Why is this drink my personal number one? It's quite simple: Once you've tossed down more than two of these infernally delicious alcoholic bombs, you'll lose pretty much all your inhibitions, but you can still fuck like a champ!

2 cL vodka
2 cL gin
2 cL rum (brown)
2 cL tequila (white)
2 cL triple sec
2 cL lemon juice
2 cL orange juice

Mix it all up together in a shaker with some ice cubes, fill into a tall glass, and top up with cola—getting your buzz on in style could hardly be easier.

5 The Sexy Cocktail: Brandy Buck
For a long time, brandy was dismissed as an old lady's tipple. But the past few years have seen a great number of wildly successful songs in the charts that sing the praises of brandy. So, there is nothing hotter than a racy brandy-based mix. It stimulates your tired taste buds—and once your tongue is properly awake, what could be more natural than to stick it down your visitor's throat?

4 cL brandy
2 cL green crème de menthe
1 cL lemon juice

Mix it up with some ice in a shaker, put some ice-cubes in a
collins glass, and pour the mixture over the top.
Top up with ginger ale, add a slice of lemon, and get ready
for a sexy evening.

4 The Fitness Cocktail: Long Distance Runner

Hot guys with sexy gym-built bodies can be terribly picky when it comes to
their eating and drinking habits—no wonder, otherwise they wouldn't have
such great bodies. But there's even a cocktail for these fussy types. Just
conjure up a fitness cocktail for him without batting an eye. You can even
add some powdered protein if he likes. In return, you could always ask him
for a bit of fitness and movement in the direction of your bedroom …

6 cL pineapple juice
1 cL passion fruit syrup
juice of half a lime

Mix it up in a shaker with some crushed ice, stick half a slice
of pineapple on the edge of the glass, drink up—and your
exhausted electrolyte supply should be nicely filled up again.
If you mention this while making the cocktail, you'll not only impress the
guy with your mixing skills but also with your profound athletic knowledge.

3 The Party Cocktail: Caipi Bull

If you're planning to take your conquest along to a wild party, I recommend
making this energy booster. It hits your bloodstream and your head straight
away—perfect as a warm-up for a long night at the club. If this
doesn't get you in the mood to party, you're probably dead.

6 cL cachaça
2 cL Red Bull

Cut up a lime and mash it up with four tablespoons of brown sugar. Then fill
up the glass with crushed ice. Pour the cachaça and Red Bull over it. The
sugar will give you a high-speed rush while the Red Bull has a more lasting
effect—let the party begin!

2 Non-Alcoholic: Virgin Mary

Of course, our list wouldn't be complete without the classic drink for the morning after. The Bloody Mary is well-known as a miracle hangover cure. However, you won't necessarily want to be glugging more alcohol after a night of doing the same. That's why I recommend a «mocktail» such as the Virgin Mary. Serve it up to your headachy conquest in bed and show him you not only have style but also class—a real gentleman!

ground black pepper
celery salt
1 dash of Tabasco
1 dash of Worcestershire sauce

Pour over ice cubes in a tall glass, add 2 cL lime cordial,
top up with tomato juice, and stir. It's best to experiment a little with the spices according to your personal taste, but it's definitely a healthy drink.

1 The Legend: Cosmopolitan

Admittedly, the Cosmopolitan definitely isn't a man's drink, but ever since *Sex and the City* made it popular again, it's become the top gay man's drink. It's definitely one worth having up your sleeve. You never know what type of guy you might pick up!

4 cL Absolut Citron
1.5 cL Cointreau
1 cL lemon juice
1 cL lime cordial
4 cL cranberry juice

Pour everything into a chilled shaker, shake it up, and pour over a few ice cubes into a tall glass. If you want to stay true to the original, you can use a cocktail glass, but that really does look a bit too girly. It's best to maintain a touch of manliness.

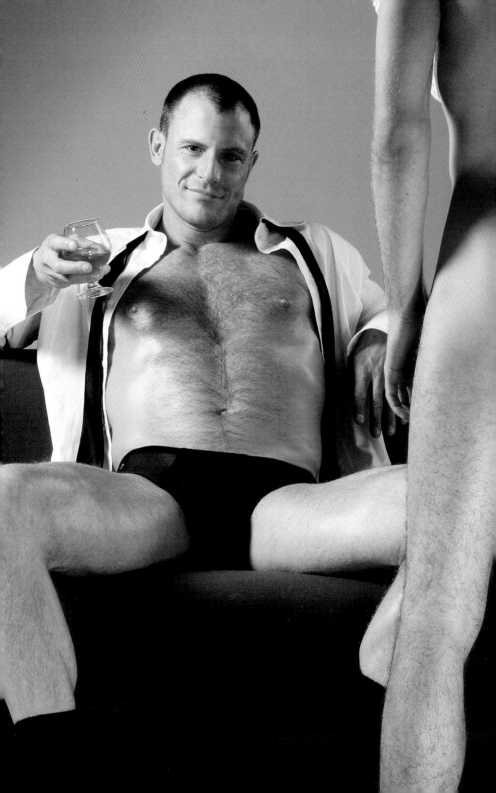

Pearls for the Pack

While I'm on the subject of alcoholic drinks, I might as well stay there for the following chapter. Slightly effeminate homos really love to clink their prosecco glasses. Real men would naturally prefer to pop real champagne corks while the more modest among us are generally happy with a glass of sparkling wine from the supermarket. Sparkling wine is simply one of the more popular gay drinks. But hardly anyone knows the difference. To combat these sinking levels of education, here is a brief overview over all the fizzy wines in our glasses.

What is sparkling wine? It's really just a blanket term for a "bottled drink with a fixed cork, pressurized by a high carbon-dioxide content." That's a very sexy description ....

Champagne

Champagne is the most chic, and as a rule most expensive, of all the sparkling wines. Its cultivation is restricted to a small area. It is pressed according to very strict rules, almost without exception from the following grapes: pinot noir for the body, pinot meunier for the fruitiness and chardonnay for its finesse. The grapes are picked by hand and the first press forms the base wine for champagne production. Up to a hundred base wines are blended before undergoing a second fermentation with yeast and sugar. If the resulting champagne is dry, it is called "brut" and contains less sugar. The tastes rage from ultra brut—super dry—to extra brut, extra sec, sec, demi sec to doux—which is very sweet. Always choose a champagne whose label gives you all the relevant details. A good choice is a "grand cru" aged for over thirty-six months and with a sugar content below fifteen grams per liter. If the label doesn't tell you any of this—don't touch it!

Sparkling Wines Made with the "Méthode Champenoise"

Of course, there a number of wines made with the same method as champagne, just not in the Champagne region. Which is why they are not allowed to call themselves that. That doesn't necessarily make them any less good, but they are frequently less expensive. The label will tell you it was made using the traditional method. A well-informed wine dealer

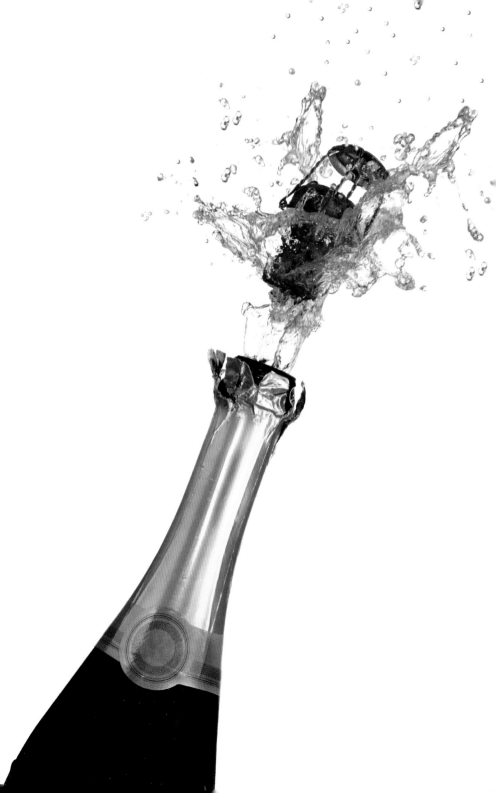

will be able to advise you. These luxury wines are available in the same bottle sizes as champagne, all of them with increasingly biblical names: from the "quart" (the piccolo) to the "imperial" (the standard size) to the "magnum" and the "Nebuchadnezzar"—the latter of which you'll only find at trashy millionaire's parties. The bottle size does have quite an effect on the taste—wine tastes better from a magnum than from a standard sized bottle. It has been out of fashion for many years, but now you should definitely order a rosé at the next important social occasion to avoid looking like an ignorant snob.

Sekt

The German or Austrian sekt is to champagne what an H&M T-shirt is to a shirt by Prada—both are produced in more or less the same fashion, but with enormous differences in the details! The ingredients and the production of sekt will never be of the same quality as champagne. But the lees—the yeast deposits that form during fermentation—are removed in the same way as its expensive brother—by disgorging. The yeast deposits that collect in the bottle neck are frozen in a clod bath, the crown cap is carefully removed, and the ice plug slides right out. A good sekt is fermented in the bottle, but most of the cheaper versions are fermented in gigantic tanks, which have a distinct effect on the quality. An even cheaper variation is to simply inject carbon dioxide into a white wine. (This revolting mess is not sold as sekt, but rather as "aerated wine.")

Marsecco

Marsecco is a speciality, pressed from the rare Marzemino grape. This sweet-tasting, blood-red grape has a bouquet of raspberries and sweet violets. Originating in Asia Minor, it spread to Venetia and the Val d'Adige in the fifteenth century, and Mozart loved the taste so much, he had the hero of his opera *Don Giovanni* call out "Eccelente Marzemino!" It's not easy to get ahold of, as it simply isn't that popular.

Prosecco

Prosecco was originally the name of a white grape, now called "Glera" which is grown in certain regions of Italy, and from which sparkling wine, aerated wine, and normal wine are produced. Vintage prosecco is protected by the "DoCG" status. Products made with the same grape but grown in other regions are now sold as Glera. The name and design of prosecco labels in particular often create the illusion of a high-quality wine. So, it's always a good idea to take a closer look or ask an expert.

Table Manners — What Every Gentleman Should Know

Nowadays, good food is an integral part of a cultivated lifestyle! I don't mean those countless cooking shows where some random person pretends to be a total gourmet, mistaking personal taste for culinary art. No, there is a discernible trend towards a cultivated enjoyment of good cuisine. And where better to enjoy this wonderful activity than over a romantic date with a gorgeous man? First you pamper your taste buds, and then everything else. Dining together can be a fantastic ritual shared by two people.

As your typical gay man is generally the gregarious type, his life will be packed with dinner parties, whether in his own home or as a guest in other people's. You'll need to learn good manners for these events. There

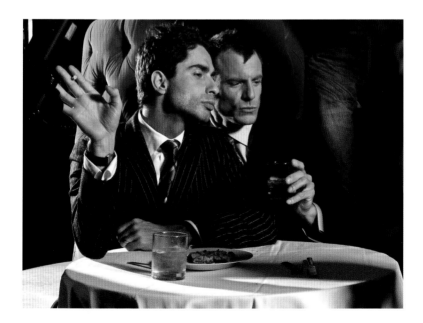

are a few rules you need to follow in order for a shared meal to become a proper gala dinner. It's not enough to gulp down your portion of meat, burp, and put your feet on the table. This will rarely impress anyone. Instead, behaving with grace and aplomb will create a much more manly impression.

So, as a real man, it can't hurt to have good table manners! This may sound a little stuffy, but Miss Manners is never wrong …

Cool Locations

If you really want to impress your date, book a table at one of the best or hippest restaurants in town. One of those places you generally only read about in the society pages in the newspaper. Do everything you can to get a good table there. Merely the fact that you're taking your guy out to this legendary place will bring him to his knees and make him open not just his heart to you. And if there happens to be a celebrity sitting at the table next to you, you'll have captured his heart. Superficial? Yeah, so what? All is fair in the war for love!

But don't let anyone see you've never been there before. Don't be too arrogant, don't get nervous or insecure. Just behave as if you were at your local bar—the only exception being that you can't choose your own table. You'll have one assigned to you! So, just wait at the entrance for someone to show you to your table. Otherwise they are guaranteed to foist off the worst possible table in you.

Knife and Fork

In a really fancy restaurant, your table will already be set with all kinds of equipment upon you arrival—so you won't be getting fresh cutlery with every new course. You will be confronted with an army of different knives, forks, spoons, and plates. This can be pretty confusing at first. But the system is really quite simple: You work your way from the outside in— that is to say, you use the outermost cutlery for the first course, the next set for the second, and so on.

No matter how delicious, please do not load up your silverware with enormous pieces. Instead, pick up small morsels of meat and vegetables. Otherwise you'll be sitting at the table chewing with your cheeks full for minutes on end—which is really bad manners and not respectful towards your date. Or were you going to talk to him with your mouth full?

Lay your knife and fork down between bites and don't get busy with them while you're still chewing. Take your time—there's no rush!

Putting down the cutlery is an art in itself. Never place your knife and fork directly on the table or half on the table and half on your plate. Lay your knife and fork across each other on your plate. This tells the waiter that you're not done with eating yet. The tines of the fork should point towards the plate.

Once you've finished eating, or have had enough, lay the knife and fork vertically sided by side on your plate, so that they both point in the same direction. This indicates to the waiter "I'm finished!" and he will clear the table.

Soup Spoon

Soup spoons are generally not placed in the respective order next to your plate with the knife and fork, but rather lined up above it. Go from top to bottom.

When eating your soup, your bowl or plate should always stay on the table. Do not grasp it in both hands to drain the last drops—even if it's really excellent soup. There are additional rules on how to eat your soup. Never spoon the soup up towards you, instead push the spoon away from the middle of the plate, away from you towards the upper edge. Then carry the spoon to your mouth—do not move your mouth towards the spoon! Never put the whole spoon in your mouth. Instead, you sip the soup from the side of the spoon—preferably without any vulgar slurping.

The Napkin

In a good restaurant, you will have a cloth napkin which you unfold and place on your lap as soon as you are seated. Never stuff it into your collar to protect your shirt from spilling—if you can't eat without spilling your food, you need to start practicing right away. (The secret of eating neatly is to only load very small morsels of food onto your fork or spoon.)

Otherwise the napkin is for you to pat your mouth on—not wipe it. It's a napkin, not a cleaning rag.

If you have to get up during your meal for any reason, excuse yourself and lay the napkin on your chair—not on the table. This tells the waiter that you'll be back. As a rule, you'll find a fresh napkin placed over the back of your chair when you get back—the waiter will have exchanged it.

When you've finished eating, please do not crumple up your napkin and dump it on your plate—that's a capital crime. Fold it up neatly and lay it on the left hand side of your plate.

Wine

On the subject of wine, in most good restaurants you will be served a different wine with every course. You can play along and drink the wine that goes with the dish. But personally, it gets on my nerves to have to constantly try a different wine, half of which I don't even like. Frequently you end up with several half-empty glasses standing around your plate—as the waiter won't take them away until they're empty—and you'll start to feel like you're sitting in a pump room. I've got into the completely acceptable habit of saying right at the start of the meal: "I'll stick to the same wine!" Then I choose a nice red wine and no longer have to worry about which glass belongs where or when and can sit back and enjoy the evening with a good drink. I also refrain from drinking the dessert wines they offer you at the end of a meal. These are usually horribly sweet and will give you a sore head the next day. But that's a matter of taste.

Apart from that, you should get into the habit of drinking a sip of water for every sip of wine you drink. That way you'll stay halfway sober and enjoy the wine instead of drinking it because you're thirsty. If you don't want any more wine, don't cover up the glass with your hand, just tell the waiter you don't want any more. Or else leave the glass alone. If it doesn't get any emptier, no one will try and top it up.

Speaking of pouring wine: It may look generous, but if you are pouring wine or champagne yourself, never fill the glass up. You should only fill it up to a third at most. Any more and it looks vulgar—as if you're implying your guests are a bunch of alcoholics.

Glasses

In most cases, there will be two or more glasses standing to the top right of your plate. The large, wide-bowled glass is for red wine. Below it, you'll find the smaller white wine glass. Next to it is the tall narrow glass for champagne and right at the bottom is your water glass. This can be an ordinary tumbler or a sturdy little wine glass. If you decide on a certain drink at the beginning of the evening and don't want to change, the surplus glasses will be cleared away.

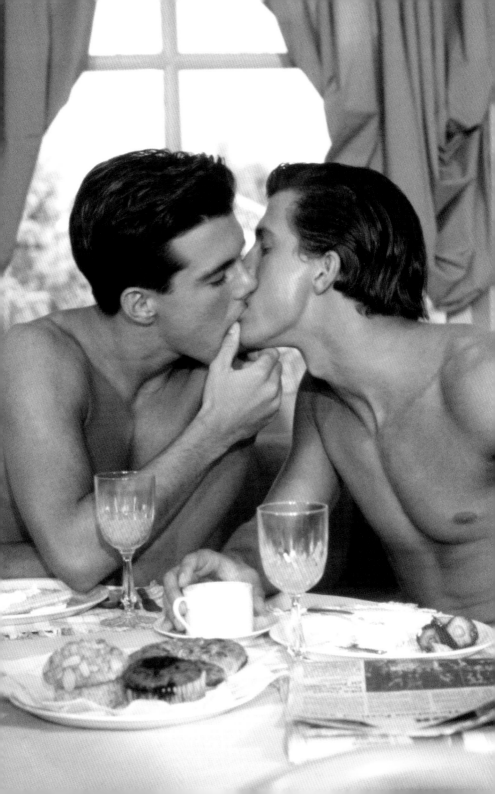

If you should ever succumb to the temptation to give a toast, never tap your glass with your spoon to get everybody's attention. Just clear your throat loudly a couple of times. The others will realize what you want soon enough. The inane habit of tapping your glass with a spoon is extremely impolite. You will very likely damage the expensive glass so that it will shatter the next time it's washed.

Seating

On the subject of seating: If it's just you and your sweetheart, there are obviously are no problems. But if the two of you have been invited to dinner within a larger circle, there are a couple of things to watch out for:

Ideally your host will have placed name cards at the respective seats to avoid confusion. Accept the seat you have been assigned and don't gripe about it. As a rule, partners are seated opposite each other, never next to each other. A good host will try and seat his guests so as to alternate between friends and strangers. Frequently enough, the place you are seated at will tell you what your host thinks of you. I take it as a personal affront if I am not seated in close proximity to my host!

When seated at the table, keep your elbows to yourself, do not gesticulate wildly, and try and keep your feet flat on the floor. Sprawling back in your chair, sticking out your legs, crossing them and inadvertently kicking other guests in the shin during dinner is generally frowned upon. What would your mother say?

Bread

In a good restaurant, you will rarely find a bread basket on the table for everyone to help themselves to. Instead a waiter will go around and offer you an assortment. Again, don't just grab a piece, tell him what you'd like. The waiter will place in your bread plate, which is to the left of the larger main plate. Bread is never cut—instead small pieces are broken off.

If there is butter for your bread, there will generally be a special butter knife placed next to your bread plate. But don't just make yourself a sandwich—spread some butter on each small piece of bread before you eat it.

Conversation

A difficult subject. The art of small-talk is essential to successfully carrying on a conversation in a larger gathering.

If you don't know all of the guests at the table, you should definitely avoid discussing politics, religion, sex, or other controversial subjects—after all, you don't want to commit a faux pas. It is not necessary to broadcast your personal opinion on every subject during dinner—sometimes silence is simply the most elegant solution!

If anyone does pipe up with an especially feeble-minded opinion, just ignore him and avoid any future contact—it's much more relaxing than submitting to an argument.

Try to divide up equally the time spent conversing with your neighbors on either side. It is terribly rude to spend the entire evening talking to one person. Of course, talking to strangers can be difficult, but remember: You are just as much a stranger to this person, and you can both spend a marvelous evening discussing the purely irrelevant. Who knows, you may suddenly realize that the person next to you is incredibly entertaining. The rule governing the time spent conversing with either neighbor is one of the most draconian of laws. It is so strict that is has given rise to the following anecdote about a well-regarded society lady, who was once seated next to her archenemy during a charity dinner. To avoid an etiquette infringement while not wanting to be obliged to speak to the persona non grata, she spent half the evening reciting the alphabet in his direction without batting an eyelid—that's real style!

A good rule of thumb in starting off a conversation with a stranger is to ask them a polite general question. Naturally this shouldn't be of an intimate nature, but rather something like: "Where are you from?" or "How do you know our host?" or "How do you like the hors d'ouevres?" Another great line is: "This is delicious wine—do you know what it is?" And then, boom! You'll spend hours chatting about trivia—after all, most people love to talk about themselves and their knowledge. You'll come across as an incredibly good, sympathetic listener.

Difficult Fare

There are a number of dishes that, while being incredibly delicious, are also very difficult to eat. Just think of the classic restaurant scene in *Pretty Woman*, where Julia Roberts struggles to eat a snail until the thing slips off the tongs and goes flying across the room. The embarrassment! To ensure that this never happens to you, here are a few of the most popular stumbling blocks in fancy cuisine:

6 If whole fruits are offered for dessert, the appropriate cutlery will already be laid out. So, you'll have to eat the fruit with a knife and fork—which really isn't easy.

TOP SIX GOURMET TRICKS

5 Artichokes are not only a fantastic beauty food, these delicious treats are also incredibly healthy. Pull off the leaves singly, holding them by the tip, and dunk the thick end into one of the dips on offer. Then suck the contents out of the fleshy end of the leaf. Lay the remains on the appropriate plate. When you've eaten all the leaves, you'll be left with the artichoke's heart—the best part! Saw off all the fine hairs with a sharp knife so that you're left with only the "meat." You can then eat that in the usual way, with a knife and fork.

4 Asparagus: Green and white asparagus are eaten differently. If you're eating the green variety, pick up a stalk in your left hand, dip it in the sauce or butter, and eat it bit by bit. If the stump is hard and woody, you don't have to eat it, just put it back on your plate. But the thicker, white asparagus is eaten in the usual way, with a knife and fork—never with your fingers.

3 Snails: these slippery bastards are decidedly difficult to eat. That's why they are generally served up with a special pair of tongs and a fork. Grab a snail with the tongs, holding on to it firmly, and use the fork to pull the meat out of the shell. Bon appétit!

2 Oysters should be slurped! Really? No! This is a common error. You can tell a real gourmet by the fact that he chews his oysters thoroughly after slurping them up. Only then will the slimy things' true taste unfold.

1 Caviar is rarely eaten on its own. Next to the small heap of fish eggs on your plate, you will generally find a number of different side dishes to eat with the caviar. These dishes range from grates egg whites and yolk to sour cream and finely chopped onions. You can tell a good caviar by the way it can be squashed with a gentle pressure between your tongue and your palate. Caviar should never be hard and "burst" in your mouth. If it tastes fishy, it's a cheap variety. Always ask for Iranian Beluga caviar. It costs a bomb, but in for a dime, in for a dollar …

General Guidelines

- If you don't like a certain dish, don't make a big deal out of it! Just pick at it elegantly so that it looks as if you'd eaten at least a little of it.
- If your food is too hot, don't blow on it to cool it off. Just wait for it to cool off on its own.
- I don't care how delicious your food is, licking your knife or plate is a total faux pas! If there is any delicious sauce left on your plate that you don't want to go to waste, mop it up with a piece of bread.
- Once you've finished your course, do not push your plate away. That's pretty impolite. Just wait for the plates to be cleared away. It really isn't that hard.
- A common mistake people often make out of insecurity, but which you should definitely avoid, is to be rude to the staff. Be polite and pleasant to your waiter. A haughty manner will only damage your standing among all those present and someone in the kitchen is guaranteed to spit in your food—no matter how fancy the restaurant.
- Whenever you take a sip of your drink, put your cutlery down first. Never hold your cutlery and your glass at the same time.
- Never outstay your welcome. Don't be the last person to leave!
- Don't leave without graciously thanking your host for the nice evening. Send him an email, or even better, a thank you letter, the next day.
- If you're unsure about a certain rule of etiquette, just discreetly watch how the other guests handle it and copy them. This is always a safe bet. Besides which, you'll come across as very polite and modest.

Breaking Up

Moving on—from everything you can do to impress the man of your dreams to a more unpleasant topic: Even the greatest love may one day come to a sticky end!

There are as many reasons to break up as there are people. Which is why I'm always annoyed when couples therapists give you the same warning signs for when a relationship is nearing its end—as some of these signs may actually signify the opposite for some couples. Besides which, actively watching for these signs can cause partners to behave in such a way that an otherwise happy relationship quickly ends up on the rocks. But let's not fool ourselves: Gay relationships are generally shorter lived than those between classic straight couples. But breaking up is still horrible every time. If you're not locked in a bitter fight to the death and you still like the guy, you won't want to hurt him. But sometimes there really is no alternative. There are five typical behavior patterns at the end of a relationship:

- the "lingerer" will feign feelings he doesn't have until he finally gets up the courage to break up with you
- the "coward" will always make you responsible and see himself as an innocent victim
- the "stylist" will actually try to find an elegant solution that is acceptable to everyone involved
- the "modernist" will break up swiftly and painlessly via email or text message
- the "attacker" will do everything in his power to start a huge fight to make it easier to split up in the midst of a feelings-storm

But there are also situations where a guy might stay with a partner who treats him badly, without really knowing why. Maybe he always lies to you or otherwise makes your life hell, but for some reason you just can't get over him—a really tricky situation. If you tell yourself: "The sex is amazing and that's why I let him treat me like dirt!" then you've only yourself to blame.

If you feel something's not quite right in your relationship for some reason, be proactive. Find out what the cause is. Otherwise your frustration will just build up and you might kill off a potentially perfect relationship in the heat of the moment just because your guy keeps on leaving the cap off the toothpaste—not very original, but sadly enough it is always the little straws of everyday life that break the emotional camel's back.

To make it easier to decide whether to keep your relationship alive, just ask yourself the following questions and then answer them honestly—no one apart from you will hear the answers. If you don't like the answers, or if they conflict with your personal philosophy of life, then it's high time for you to seriously reconsider your relationship and possibly keep your eyes open for someone new.

Relationship Red Flags

If you've noticed that there are certain topics or problems within your relationship that you can't discuss without causing an enormous fight or hurt feelings, that should be your first red flag. You need to find a way out of these kinds of situations as quickly as possible, otherwise you'll be carrying the conflict around inside you for a long time, and that does no one any good!

- Has your partner frequently hurt or disappointed you?
- Do you get the feeling your partner doesn't care about you and your interests?
- Do you get the feeling he might be selfish?
- Do you feel manipulated by your partner?
- Can he admit to mistakes and apologize for them?
- Can he forgive you?
- Can he accept compromises in the small things in life?
- Are you sometimes afraid of him when he is angry?
- How does he treat other people when he's angry?
- Has he ever threatened or even hit you?
- Does he listen to what you want?
- Do you trust him?
- Is he honest and reliable?
- Does he have a drug or alcohol problem?
- Does he add to the problems in your life or does he make them easier?
- Are you both proud of being seen together?

If doesn't matter whether or not your fears are well founded. They are true for you and there is a reason for this. Something isn't working for you and you need to determine the cause.

Maybe he's kind and considerate to you, but you keep seeing him treat other people badly. See that as a warning that you might be one of these "other people" for him, too, someday.

If you notice he has trouble fulfilling his obligations at work, towards friends or the gym, he might well stop fulfilling his obligations towards you, despite his promises of undying faithfulness.

You should also be suspicious if you never get to meet his friends and family. This may well mean he doesn't want to be seen with you.

How he behaves during conflicts is another sign of how he will behave towards you in the future—this phenomenon has been the subject of much research and is scientifically proven. If you realize early on in your relationship that he has a tendency towards violence, be extremely careful. He may take his anger out on objects at first, but over time, he may well lose his regard for you as well. Be proactive here and insist that he get treatment.

Pay attention to how he talks about his exes. This is always a very clear sign of how he behaves towards other people in general.

And this may sound brutal, but if you find out he has problems with drugs or alcohol, break up with him right away. Don't believe in the myth of love conquering all. You are not a doctor and you shouldn't be one in your relationship. Love cannot cure an addiction. Either he seeks treatment or you're out of there. Right away!

But you don't always have to break up right away. If the two of you have good communication and you both want to save the relationship, seek help from a couples therapist or a couples coach. These days, you can find a number of therapists that specialize in gay couples—and often enough, a few small changes in everyday life can make a gay marriage a happy one. I'm speaking from experience on two counts: On the one hand, a coach has helped me put my own relationship put back on its feet, and on the other, I have seen many quarreling couples leave my office, happy once more, in the course of my own work as a coach.

If nothing helps: Make a radical break!

Break up! No ifs, ands, or buts! Be direct, consistent, and honest. Draw the line and don't use the word "but" when making and explaining your

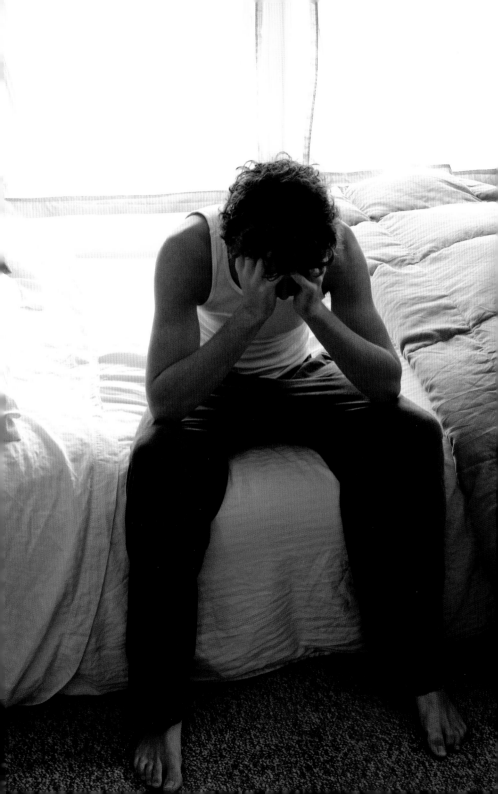

decision. You can only make this breakup halfway short and painless for both of you if you're totally clear with yourself and your actions and can convey this. Don't play the blame game. Just talk about how you feel, without laying the blame on anyone. You don't have to explain yourself! Your goal should be to end something well, not to embark on a campaign of revenge. Keep your dignity and let him keep his! Do not break up via text message or any other cowardly method. Man up!

The best breakup location is on neutral ground, somewhere a noisy fight or physical altercation will be difficult. So, don't do it at his home or

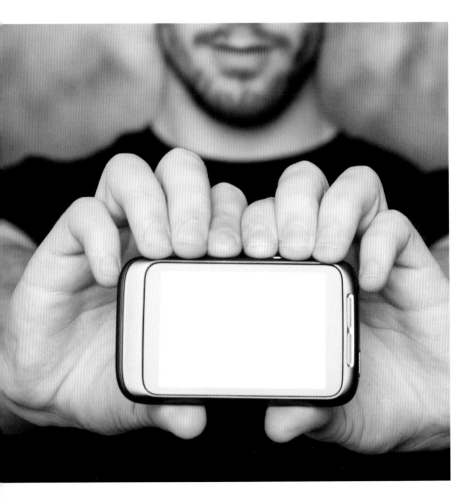

yours. Also, after breaking up, avoid going to any of the places the two of you used to frequent together, such as the gym, bars, or the supermarket. Be the bigger person and put yourself out a bit to make the breakup easier for both of you.

Most important of all: do not have "break-up-sex"—the recidivism rate following this is very high and it will be even harder to break up next time.

See the end of your relationship as an opportunity! The end is always the beginning of something new.

New adventures await you. But don't be too desperate to find a new partner right away. Get to know yourself as a single person. Fulfill your inner dreams. Maybe there's a sport you've always wanted to learn, a place you've always wanted to visit, or maybe you just need to spend a weekend binge-watching DVDs—now you'll finally have the time to do everything that makes you feel good!

P.S. If your guy tries to blackmail you in any way, such as "I'll kill myself if you leave me," leave immediately. Do not turn back! Leave him standing there or hang up. Signalize very clearly that he's well out of order. Think about what he's trying to do to you—blackmailing you into loving him. That should make you angry enough to open the window yourself and invite him to jump out of it! If you have any serious concerns, call his friends or his family and ask them to keep an eye on him. But expressly forbid them from telling him to contact you.

Breaking Up Via Text Message

Even with the best intentions, breaking up can go horribly wrong and sometimes nothing works smoothly and elegantly enough for both parties to emerge from the situation without being injured psychologically. Sometimes you'll have to end a relationship in self-defense because your partner is a real asshole and you unfortunately noticed too late.

The best way to blow off a guy like that is—and this is the exception to the rule—by sending an obnoxious text message! Thanks to a digital slap in the face you won't have to see his dumb face ever again. If you're so angry at this guy that you can't even find the right words, here are my personal top ten "Game Over" texts:

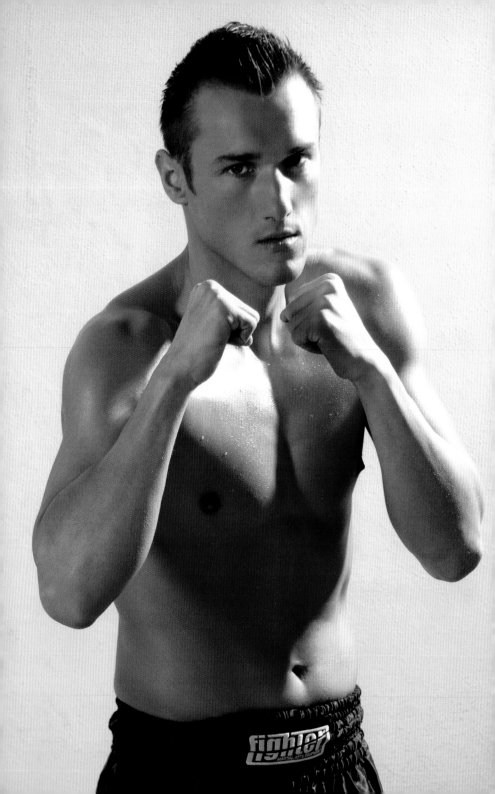

**TOP TEN
THE END
VIA TEXT**

10 I forgot about myself because I loved you. Now I'm forgetting about you because I love myself!

9 I'll never forget the first time we met, but I'll keep trying.

8 I don't know how to live without you. But tomorrow, it's time to find out.

7 You know how much I love good company. Which is I won't be seeing you anymore. Bye!

6 Roses are red violets are blue, I'd rather be dead than go on seeing you!

5 Your body is perfect, your ass is hot and I love your personality! … Shit. Wrong number!

4 If your dick were any shorter, it would be an internal organ! And I'm no internist! Bye!

3 I was going to tell you over the phone. But that wouldn't be very nice. That would be too easy, too tactless. Let me give it to you in writing instead: It's over!

2 Sorry, I never realized just how ugly you are!

1 I've already told a lot of people to kiss my rosy red ass. Today is your day!

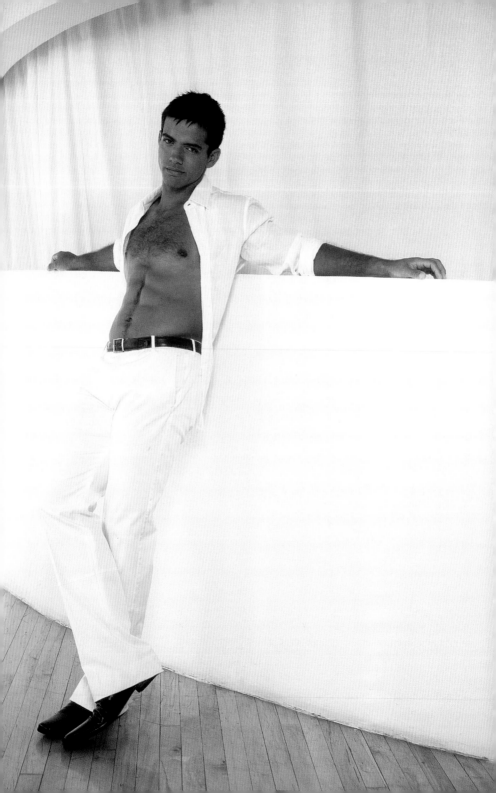

Your Apartment

One of the most intimate moments in a gay man's life is when he welcomes a new acquaintance into his apartment for the first time—sex is a walk in the park compared to this. Our homes say much more about us than we may want them to. Whether it's messy or painfully neat, furnished in style or with a couple of orange crates, art prints on the wall, or just a few torn-out photos of naked men—your own apartment affords other people a direct look into the depths of your soul. It's the same for gay and straight men. While women frequently obscure any discernable individual touches behind piles of ornaments and other tchotchkes, the average man lays bare the very core of his being.

Gay apartments play such a special role that there are already countless Web sites online dedicated to exposing the more bizarre furnishing accidents revealed by gay men in their online dating profiles. A sling, for instance, hanging next to a withered ficus plant on an imitation Roman pedestal, while in the background, thick velvet curtains are twined dramatically around a curtain rod. Another popular feature seems to be flea-bitten couches and armchairs in all the colors of vomit, squeezed into a studio apartment in front of the Early Colonial sideboard inherited from Grandma, above them a cheesy chandelier draped with red fabric panels—all this apparently occurs so frequently, one might be tempted to think that the average gay man sees himself with a regal calling, rather than committing to a merely bourgeois lifestyle. But it does get better. According to a recent survey, 17.3 percent of all gay men say that their apartments are a status symbol and that they spend a disproportionate amount of money on them.

According to this survey, the perfect gay apartment should boast large rooms, well-lit rooms, high ceilings, and an Internet connection. And while straight men don't seem to care either way, gay men would like their dream apartment to be situated in the inner city, not too far from a few good restaurants and bars, and easy to reach by public transport. Heteros' only real desire is for a good infrastructure for their kids, while gay men, for obvious reasons, tend to ignore this point.

Furnishings should reflect a certain status. Among gay men, the following items, or at least copies of the same, are popular; the "Barcelona chair" by Ludwig Mies van der Rohe and Lilly Reich or Charles Eames's "Lounge chair"—you'll find these objects in pretty much every well-equipped gay home.

A Brief Guide to Furnishing Your Chic Gay Apartment

Since not everyone was born the perfect interior designer, here's a handy guide so that every gorgeous man can be shown to the best advantage in his even more gorgeous apartment.

Basic Rule: A masculine apartment should always be decorated with clear structures in mind. Anything contorted or cluttered tends to be seen as feminine.

Once you've left college—or at the very latest, once you discover your first gray hairs—it's time to ditch the furniture from your childhood. Nothing screams immaturity louder than sagging bedsprings, Mom's old kitchen furnishings, or a completely threadbare sofa. If you don't respect your surroundings, you're implying that you don't respect yourself.

If you furnish your apartment straight out of a furnishing catalogue, you won't ever develop your own original style—and that's what decorating your apartment is about. You need to be able to see yourself in your own home. Let yourself be inspired, but don't just copy.

Buying furniture from a cheap warehouse saves you money and looks good at a first glance, but few people know what they'll be taking home with them. The same nasty chemicals that have gone into tanning the leather on your sofa will also turn up in your plyboard closet. And to cap it all off, you'll also have supported child labor and unfair wages with your miserliness. So, stop complaining about all the misery in world and start to live accordingly.

Too much is definitely too much! Gay men in particular tend to hopelessly overfurnish their apartments—especially if they don't have that much room. Instead, make sure there is enough space to breathe in your home.

Stick with plain, darker colors—these are more masculine. Use art prints on the walls or small ornaments to create dashes of color. Don't get too experimental with color combinations that might drive the calmest personalities straight into the psychiatric ward.

Men need comfortable apartments. When choosing furniture, make sure you can actually live with it. A hyper-modernist kitchen chair may look incredibly stylish, but you risk bruising your guests' backsides because the thing is so damn uncomfortable. Comfort should be your first priority!

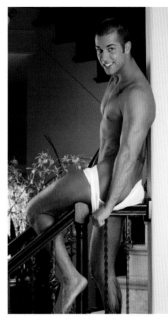

Get yourself some curtains or shades. In large cities in particular there is a trend towards the "open window." You can watch pretty much the entire neighborhood performing the most embarrassingly intimate activities as nobody seems to have curtains anymore. But curtains will warm the soul of your apartment. Of course, you should steer clear of old-fashioned lace curtains. Instead, get yourself a set of padded, opaque curtains, hung generously, so that they don't look like an economy model.

Work on your lighting. If your budget won't allow for sophisticated lighting, here's a visual trick: Get rid of the overhead light and use floor and table lamps to create an elegant atmosphere. This will make even the barest room look like a design temple.

Get rid of all your posters of muscular men holding car tires or babies in their arms. The classic homo posters are at least twenty years past their expiration date. Don't choose your wall decorations according to mass appeal. Instead hang up the stuff that really touches your soul.

Make sure your kitchen is well-equipped, even if you don't cook that much or that well. Cooking has become such a popular pastime that the next guy you meet is guaranteed to be delighted to find everything he needs in your kitchen to conjure up the most fabulous meals for you.

What Effect Do Colors Have in Your Apartment?

Ever since Ty Pennington trundled through a series of badly furnished homes on U.S. television, leaving gaudy splashes of color on one wall after the next, half the nation has been attempting to turn their homes into a box of water paints. Color me beautiful has given way to color me insane. First of all, all the cheaply refurnished apartments you see on reality design shows will look totally shabby in about two months' time, and secondly, it is catastrophically naive to believe that any family could ever lead a harmonious life in a bright red kitchen. Colors affect us more than we would like. This has been proven in a number of scientific studies.

I speak from personal experience. In a rush of creative insanity, I once made the ill-advised decision to paint my kitchen bright green—who would ever be able to resist that healthy fresh color? Wrong call! As soon as I switched on the kitchen light, the green walls threw an unwholesome gleam onto the faces of all the hapless people in the room so that they resembled a collection of decomposing corpses. The paint didn't stay up for long, and no wonder.

Which is why I'm giving you this overview of colors and their effects, to help you make a more informed decision.

Red is the color of love and passion, but you have to get the shade exactly right and only apply it in homeopathic doses. For as a rule, red causes aggression and creates tension. Besides which, the color red stimulates the appetite and will ruin your vacation figure. Instead of painting the walls red, try using red lighting. That will make you hungry—not just for heavy food, but for hot sex as well!

Yellow can signalize golden showers to those in the know, but in your apartment it can stand for joy and optimism. Yellow can also calm anxiety and depression and have a detoxifying effect—but only if you use uncontaminated organic paint. Bright yellow will make small rooms seem larger and stimulate concentration and creativity—the ideal color for your study.

Dark green has a soothing effect. Shades of green can even alleviate anger and lovesickness. So, it's a good idea to establish a green corner somewhere in your apartment. You can also add some green to your home by buying a few plants.

Blue is one of the more intense colors you can use in your home. A dark Yves Klein shade of blue will create an atmosphere of pleasant melancholy, while a pale sky blue will bring lightness to a room. It's a good color for your bedroom, as blue can combat sleep disorders and encourage mental clarity.

Gray is the new white. Light gray is the perfect color for your walls, radiating elegant restraint and classiness. But steer clear of boring mousy shades. It's best to get an expert to advise you on picking the perfect shade. Combined with white ceilings, gray can look positively regal.

Brown is the ideal color for every apartment. It is a calm, earthy color and it radiates safety. It is used in color therapy to treat balance disorders. But not the classic seventies turd color—I'm talking about a modern, elegant brown. If you're still dubious, remember that ever since 2009, brown is the color of the future for the automobile industry. I'm talking about a shade of brown closer to coffee than mud.

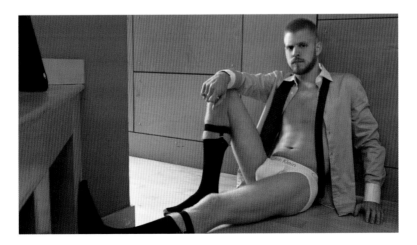

Lie Down! – Choosing the Right Mattress

We spend nearly a third of our lives in bed—and that's just the time spent actually sleeping in bed. But in many gay households, the bedroom and the bed in particular are subject to neglect. While the kitchen is equipped like that of a three-star restaurant and the living room is furnished with chic chairs and couches and a gigantic flat-screen TV, the bedroom is home to an ancient mattress slumped hopelessly over a cheap wooden frame from a cheap Swedish furniture store. But true style is not revealed in single pieces of furniture showcased in your apartment, but rather in the details—being conscious of quality and being prepared to look after oneself. And what better place to do that than in bed? Not only because that's the place where you succumb to the carnal pleasures, but also because sleeping well is essential for your physical and mental well-being. If you sleep badly, your concentration suffers, your mood suffers, and you catch cold more easily. While you're asleep, your body uses the time to fight disease, your brain processes the impressions the day has left, and the muscles you have built up at the gym have time to grow. Besides which, studies have shown that sleep deprivation can make you fat!

Many people just think the old mattress they've been hauling around with them for years will still do just fine. But that's only because they've never heard that every person loses about 1.5 milligrams of dead skin per night. This feeds the approximately 10,000 mites that live in your mattress. Just the thought of all those billions of mites I've been feeding with my own and other people's skin by the pound makes me feel nauseous.

Which is why I make sure to regularly buy a new—high-quality—mattress. Experts recommend buying a new one every eight to ten years.

How to Choose the Right Mattress
Here are a few established rules on buying an affordable mattress that will make your dreams so much sweeter.

Going to a specialty store is a must, for without an expert's advice and without trying it out, you'll end up with a mattress about as comfortable as a fakir's bed of nails. Individual mattress choice will vary according to build, weight, and any health problems you may have.

The first point to consider is the mattress' firmness. Medical researchers tested different sleeping positions on dummies and found out that it is extremely important for the mattress to yield in the right places. A too firm mattress will not release pressure from your skeletal structure, causing tension.

A healthy spine is naturally shaped like a double S, forming a straight line from top to bottom. According to your sleeping position therefore, your mattress should be built so that the shoulders and pelvis of side-sleepers, for instance, can sink into the mattress deeply enough for this line to be formed by itself.

The claim that it is healthier to lie on a hard surface has been disproved. A hard surface will only benefit those suffering from a slipped disk.

For your guidance, there are three degrees of firmness:
- soft for people weighing up to 130 pounds
- medium for people weighing up to 180 pounds
- for all the heavier guys: firm for anyone over 180 pounds

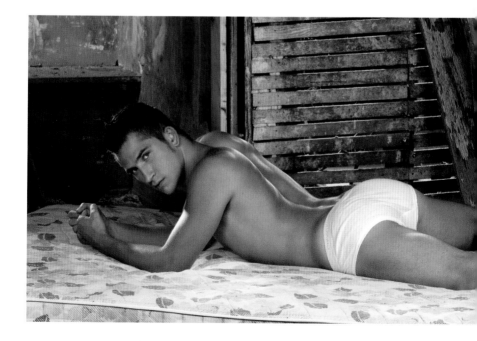

The thickness also plays an important part. The thicker a mattress is, the less the risk of compression. This is when the mattress' filling can no longer yield to the weight of the body lying on it. A mattress should be at least six inches thick, and while we're speaking of measurements, the height of the mattress is also important. Your sleeping position should be at least twenty-three inches above the floor, as the air in the room below this level is a lot less fresh and contains a higher amount of allergens and bacteria. Fortunately, the low-level futon trend is now a thing of the past.

The mattress should be divided up into different zones so that it can adapt itself perfectly to your body via different levels of firmness. Ideally, you would insist on a "cube cut" instead of a "wave cut" and really impress your salesperson! But you can only find out what the ideal distribution for you is by trying it out! Time and patience are indispensable!

Inner spring mattresses are the traditional classic. They offer the best ventilation, good support, and are relatively inexpensive. There are some cheaper models on the market, but you should avoid those. The weight is unevenly distributed over the springs in cheap mattresses and will quickly lead to the dreaded "saggy mattress," not to mention the tension in your body caused by its being forced to lie in an unnatural position. Individual springs can lose their shape or rust, deforming the other neighboring springs as well.

So, never buy Bonnell or continuous coil mattresses. Pocket spring mattresses are an excellent, if somewhat more expensive, alternative. Get a five-coil pocket spring mattress and make sure there are upholstery layers attached, so that you don't feel every single coil. The best upholstery starts at one inch.

Make sure to check the bulk density as well. This should not be less than thirty. The metal coils should also be "grounded" to prevent them from creating electrosmog and a magnetic field, which can cause sleep disorders and tension in many sleepers.

Even at the lower end of the price range, latex mattresses are a more expensive alternative. While they cost upwards of $250, they are incredibly comfortable as they automatically adjust to your body and are very hygienic. The main disadvantage is that they are relatively air-tight. This will make you sweat more readily in your sleep. To make things worse, your sweat will not be absorbed by the mattress but can only evaporate into the air—so in the warmer months you'll be lying in a revolting puddle.

Guys who go in for a lot of mattress tango-ing should avoid this type, as all kinds of bacteria can grow in the fluids that collect there. Besides which, the damn things are incredibly heavy! It is almost impossible to move one of these latex monsters without help—making every move an agony.

Foam mattresses are a good alternative—effective and relatively inexpensive. They are light and well-ventilated while adjusting well to your body. But make sure that the core of your foam mattress is at least five inches thick and has a bulk density of more than forty.

As a guideline: You should plan to spend at least $600 on a new mattress. This may sound like a lot, but it will guarantee you sleep well for many years. The motto—the more expensive the better—certainly holds true for mattresses.

By the way, it's not enough to just buy a new mattress. You should also buy a new bed base to fit your new mattress. Otherwise you'll lose all the benefits of having a good mattress.

What Makes a Good Bed Base?

It should have at least twenty-eight sprung slats, each of them at least 1.5 inches wide. These should be glued at six points, and the gap between them should be no more than 1.5 inches wide. The slats should be connected with a central strap. Caution: Do not buy a slatted base made of softwood, pine, or larch wood. Beech wood slats are much better! Also make sure there is a functional shoulder zone as well as an adjustable pelvis and back zone.

If all these requirements are met, nothing will stand in the way of a new sensational sleeping experience. The first nights will be rather uncomfortable, as upgrading from an old foam mat to a high-quality mattress means your body will have to learn how to lie properly again. But you will soon come to appreciate the positive effects of your new mattress, the same as every willing visitor to your brand new bed!

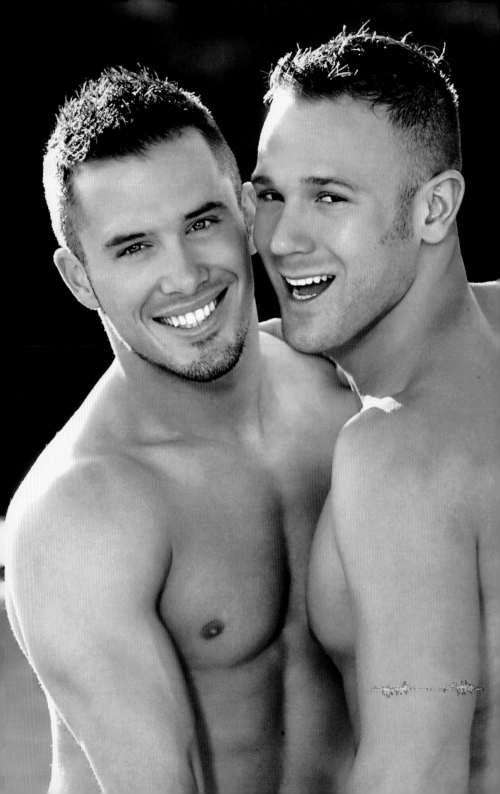

Thanks

It is patently clear that, in spite of my experi-
ence as a lifestyle writer and life coach, I could
never have written this book alone! I'll give a
polite curtsey at this point and say thank you
to my husband, who, years ago, had to forcibly
open my eyes to the benefits of the really good
life—thank you, darling! I could never have
done it without you!

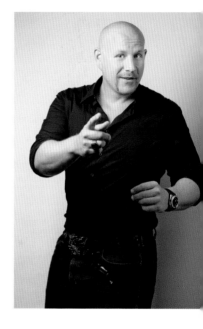

Many, many thanks to the world's best trainer:
Thomas Wenzl! There'll be much more to come!
And many thanks to Susanne Pajunk, who
forgave even my worst spelling goofs with a
charming smile!

Thank you, too, to Peter Rehberg—it's been a
long while, but this book would not have been
written without him!

And thanks a million to all those lovely boys who helped with this book—
you know who you are!

Last but not least, thank you to all the girls in the many, many agencies
with whom I worked on all those super beauty and lifestyle topics in the
past years! You are all wonderful!

P.S. Before I forget—thank you for buying this book. I hope you have enjoyed reading it as much as I enjoyed writing it! Thanks—hugs and kisses!

Sex Made Better … and Better

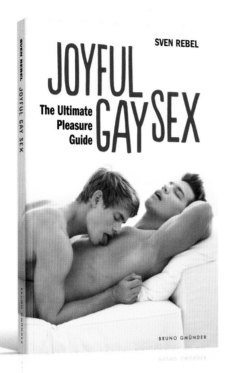

Sven Rebel
JOYFUL GAY SEX
The Ultimate Pleasure Guide
192 pages, softcover,
full color
14 x 21 cm, 5½ x 8¼"
ISBN 978-3-86787-601-8
US$ 24.99 / € 21,95

Every generation discovers gay sex in its own way: new sex symbols, styles and fetishes appear and take the place of old ones; familiar sex practices become less popular , while people love each other in exciting new ways. From the tried and true to the exotic and adventurous, this book offers expert tips and nexpected tricks to make gay sex an even more joyful experience.

Guidebooks for the Curious and Adventurous

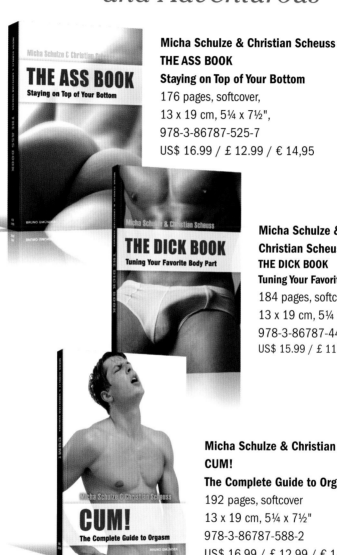

Micha Schulze & Christian Scheuss
THE ASS BOOK
Staying on Top of Your Bottom
176 pages, softcover,
13 x 19 cm, 5¼ x 7½",
978-3-86787-525-7
US$ 16.99 / £ 12.99 / € 14,95

Micha Schulze &
Christian Scheuss
THE DICK BOOK
Tuning Your Favorite Body Part
184 pages, softcover,
13 x 19 cm, 5¼ x 7½"
978-3-86787-446-5
US$ 15.99 / £ 11.99 / € 14,95

Micha Schulze & Christian Scheuss
CUM!
The Complete Guide to Orgasm
192 pages, softcover
13 x 19 cm, 5¼ x 7½"
978-3-86787-588-2
US$ 16.99 / £ 12,99 / € 14,95

Gay Erotica at Its Best

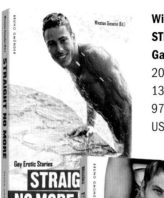

Winston Gieseke (Ed.)
STRAIGHT NO MORE
Gay Erotic Stories
208 pages, softcover,
13 x 19 cm, 5¼ x 7½",
978-3-86787-607-0
US$ 17.99 / £ 11.99 / € 16,95

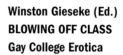

Winston Gieseke (Ed.)
BLOWING OFF CLASS
Gay College Erotica
208 pages, softcover
13 x 19 cm, 5¼ x 7½"
978-3-86787-686-5
US$ 17.99 / £ 11.99 / € 15,95

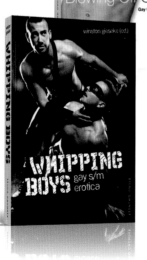

Winston Gieseke (Ed.)
WHIPPING BOYS
Gay S/M Erotica
208 pages, softcover
13 x 19 cm, 5¼ x 7½"
978-3-86787-689-6
US$ 17.99 / £ 11.99 / € 15,95

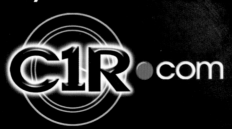

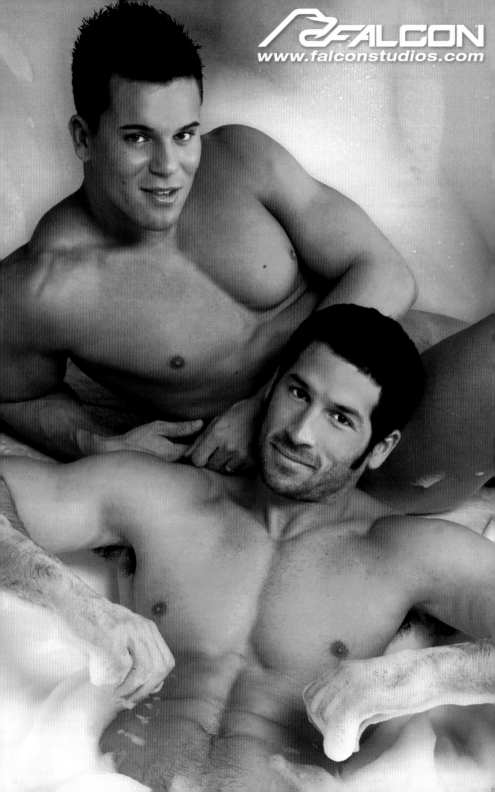

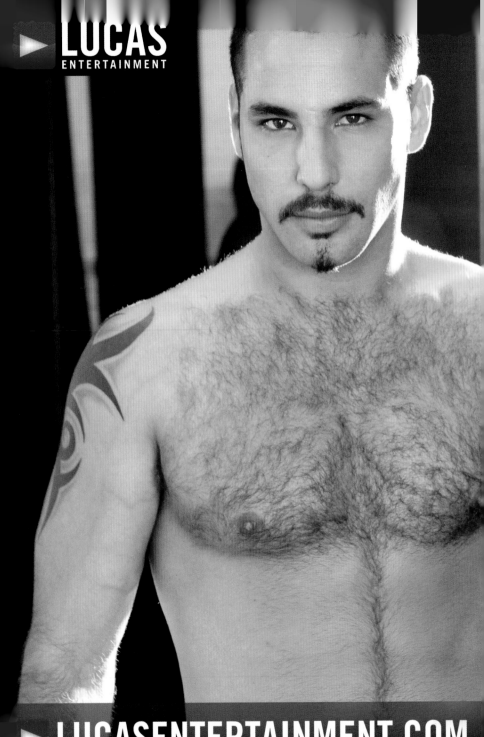